TABLE OF CONTENTS

Rehabilitation in Managed Care
Controlling Cost
Ensuring Quality

Chris Hagen, PhD, SLP
Director
Rehab Solutions Inc.
Escondido, California

AN ASPEN PUBLICATION®
Aspen Publishers, Inc.
Gaithersburg, Maryland
1999

The author has made every effort to ensure the accuracy of the information herein. However, appropriate information sources should be consulted, especially for new or unfamiliar procedures. It is the responsibility of every practitioner to evaluate the appropriateness of a particular opinion in the context of actual clinical situations and with due considerations to new developments. The author, editors, and the publisher cannot be held responsible for any typographical or other errors found in this book.

Library of Congress Cataloging-in-Publication Data

Hagen, Chris.
Rehabilitation in managed care: controlling cost,
ensuring quality / Chris Hagen.
Includes bibliographical references and index.
ISBN 0-8342-0923-3
1. Managed care plans (Medical care)—Patients—Care.
2. Managed care plans (Medical care)—Economic aspects.
3. Managed care plans (Medical care)—Quality control.
4. Medical rehabilitation.
I. Title.
RA413.H34   1999
362.1'04258—dc21
99-12291
CIP

Orders: (800) 638-8437
Customer Service: (800) 234-1660

About Aspen Publishers • For more than 35 years, Aspen has been a leading professional publisher in a variety of disciplines. Aspen's vast information resources are available in both print and electronic formats. We are committed to providing the highest quality information available in the most appropriate format for our customers. Visit Aspen's Internet site for more information resources, directories, articles, and a searchable version of Aspen's full catalog, including the most recent publications: **http://www.aspenpublishers.com**
Aspen Publishers, Inc. • The hallmark of quality in publishing
Member of the worldwide Wolters Kluwer group.

Editorial Services: Kathy Litzenberg
Library of Congress Catalog Card Number: 99-12291
ISBN: 0-8342-0923-3

Printed in the United States of America

1 2 3 4 5

PREFACE

The financing of rehabilitation is rapidly and irrevocably changing from a fee-for-service and cost-plus method of payment to the capitated method of managed care. This change is also bringing a significant change in the role of the therapist. In the past, the responsibilities of the therapist included evaluating the client and managing his or her course of rehabilitation to achieve the best possible outcome. Managing the cost of rehabilitation was seen as the responsibility of "administration." However, as rehabilitation moves into the era of managed care, the roles and responsibilities of the therapist will expand beyond the purely clinical domain. They will not only entail clinical excellence but also the ability to exert fiscal control over limited resources. Good job performance will not simply be the achievement of the best outcome. It will be achieving the best outcome for the least cost.

The purpose of this book is to provide therapists and their managers with a clinical decision-making model, a decision-making system, and the tools to move from the historical role of therapist to today's role of a clinical case manager. The objective of the book is to provide a means by which the therapist can manage both the quality and cost of services while simultaneously preserving professional ethics, individualized client care, and professional identity. Each chapter of this book is directed toward the attainment of this objective.

Chapter 1 is designed to increase the reader's understanding of the goal of managed care and why the financing of health care has to move away from the fee-for-service method of payment to the managed care method of payment. This chapter also provides definitions of key managed care terms. To understand why and how the fiscal constraints that are placed on the provider of service by the payer affect clinical decision making, the therapist must have at least a rudimentary knowledge of the financial side of rehabilitation. Chapter 2 presents basic information about the business side of rehabilitation. It covers the equation between revenue and expenses in both the nonprofit and for-profit environments. The difference between fee for service, per diem, capitated rates, and shared risk is discussed. Finally, the purposes and functions of managed care organizations, indemnity insurance, Medicare, and Medicaid are reviewed. Chapters 1 and 2 lay the foundation as to *why* the therapist's role and responsibilities must now expand to those of a clinical case manager. Chapter 3 defines *what* clinical resources must be managed. Chapters 4 and 5 show the therapist *how* to manage those resources. They present a clinical decision-making model, system, and tools that can be used to manage cost through incisive clinical decision making. Chapter 6 focuses on the critical role the family plays in attaining the most appropriate outcome in the least amount of time and the durability of that outcome after the client is discharged from rehabilitation.

Making hard clinical decisions, such as which disciplines are more important than others given the constraints imposed by a client's financial resources or how the disciplines should be sequenced across time to most effectively and cost efficiently meet a client's needs, requires a self-managed rehabilitation team. Chapter 7 provides methods that will assist a multidisciplinary team to move past discipline boundaries in their clinical decision-making process and evolve into a self-managed rehabilitation team. Documentation is the cornerstone of both good clinical management and reimbursement. Chapter 8 presents practical documentation methods that will produce the type of clear and objective information required for sound clinical decision making and appropriate reimbursement.

ACKNOWLEDGMENTS

I thank my wonderful wife for her unflagging support and assiduous proofreading of each chapter. I am also deeply indebted to my "volunteer" editor Dr. Kay Butler whose comments, questions, and suggestions were extremely helpful. Finally, I thank my good friend and colleague, Mary Foto, OT, for her invaluable help with the ever changing and unfolding Medicare information.

CHAPTER 1

Managed Care: Where Did It Come from, What Is It, and Why Should I Care?

KEY POINTS

- The changes in our health care delivery system are driven by the cost of health care.

- Managed care integrates clinical decisions and cost decisions.

- Under managed care, provider profitability will be found more in cost containment than in generating revenue.

- Managed care will change the traditional roles and responsibilities of the therapist.

Tremendous changes have occurred in our health care delivery system, changes that will significantly alter therapists' historical manner of providing their services. The vehicle for this change is called "managed care." Managed care is a general term that refers to any organization that directs access to health care services to ensure that its clients receive high quality of care in a cost-effective manner. In the past, there was no linkage between those responsible for the payment for health care services and those who provided them. Managed care organizations (MCOs) have changed this historical relationship between payer and provider. They have integrated and centralized the control of both the financing and delivery of health care services.[1] They are directly involved in the client's choice of service providers as well as the type of service that is provided. As a result, the therapist is no longer the sole clinical decision maker regarding the type, frequency, and/or duration of the services provided. The soaring costs of health care have fueled this change.[2] In 1992, health care expenditures were 14 percent of the gross domestic product, or $835.5 billion. This means roughly that about $3,200 were spent on health care for each American that year.[3] At the same time, employers have experienced an ever escalating increase in the cost of employee health care benefits. In 1990, they paid $174 billion in employee premiums, an amount almost equal to their net profits.[4] "Cost shifting" by providers created another source for the increasing costs of health care. Medicare diagnosis-related groups (DRGs), limits imposed by the Tax Equity and Fiscal Responsibility Act (TEFRA, Public Law 97-248 of 1982), and Medicaid's schedule of maximum allowances placed a cap on provider revenue, significantly reducing provider profitability when serving these populations. To continue to serve the Medicare and Medicaid populations and maintain profitability, providers "shifted" their costs to the private pay sector. They increased the fees for their services. While Medicare and Medicaid would only pay preestablished rates, not the amount charged, the private insurance companies, employers, and individuals did pay the actual amount charged. Thus, the providers maintained their ability to remain profitable by shifting the cost of service delivery that was not covered for their Medicare and Medicaid patients to the "private pay" patients. As a result, the cost of health care continued to spiral out of control.

Today, Americans find that their health care consumption is being severely restrained, due primarily to the absence of cost control over the past 30 years. Prior to the late 1950s, the individual was the primary purchaser of health care services. Paying out of your own pocket provides a natural incentive to use such services judiciously. This natural restraint on health care consumption began to change in the 1960s, a time when insurance companies, employers, and the federal government rapidly replaced individuals as the major purchasers of health care services. Employers offered health care coverage as an employee benefit and purchased health insurance plans from insurance companies. Simultaneously, there was a growing increase in the number of individuals who directly purchased health care insurance. During this same era, the federal goverment established the Medicare and Medicaid programs. Their establishment ushered in an era of abundant and unlimited access to health care. From a sociological perspective, this was a major advancement in the individual's quality of life. Absent any spending controls or restraints, however, this was also the beginning of our current economic dilemma regarding health care costs. The 1960s produced a health care system in which there was unlimited demand for services and an unlimited supply. As long as the individual did not have to pay directly for services, there was no incentive to use them judiciously. Similarly, as long as the provider was the sole decision maker regarding the type, frequency, and duration of services and was paid in full for services no matter what their cost, there was no incentive to develop more efficient and less costly service delivery systems. In effect, this health care environment promoted overutilization of health care services.[5] As this resource consumption went unchecked, the insurance companies found that they were paying more for the services than the insurance premiums they were collecting. Meanwhile, the demand for services through the Medicare and Medicaid programs began to outgrow their level of funding. As service demands increased, health care providers, including physicians, increased their fees; insurance companies raised the premiums charged to the employers; and federal and state governments allocated more tax dollars to health care. Over time, insurance company and employer profits declined and citizens increasingly raised questions about a governmental health care system that had no way of controlling its consumption of taxpayer dollars.

As employer and insurance company profits continued to decline and the cost of the Medicare and Medicaid programs mushroomed, the push for cost controls began in earnest. The first attempts at cost control focused solely on what insurance companies perceived as financial incentives that would slow down the individual's consumption of services. The insurance industry instituted a system that required enrollees to pay a specified amount of money out of their own pocket—a deductible—before the insurance plan would pay for any services. When this did not achieve the desired results, they added a co-payment requirement in which the consumer pays a percentage of the service provider's charges. Employers responded to the situation by shifting a portion of their health care benefit costs to their employees by asking them to pay for a portion of their insurance premium and increasing their deductibles. In 1982, Congress passed the Tax Equity and Fiscal Responsibility Act (Public Law 97-248). A portion of that law, commonly referred to as TEFRA, was the first step toward trying to control the costs of inpatient rehabilitation services provided to Medicare beneficiaries. Historically, providers of inpatient rehabilitation services had been reimbursed on the basis of their "reasonable" costs for providing the services. TEFRA imposed an annual maximum cost, called the TEFRA limit, that the Health Care Financing Administration (HCFA) would pay for inpatient rehabilitation services.[6] During this same time period, state governments set fees (i.e., the schedule of maximum allowances) that they would pay for Medicaid services. In essence, the TEFRA limit and the schedule of maximum allowances were the first attempts to create a prospective payment system (PPS) for rehabilitation services; a payment system in which the amount that will be paid is determined before the services are rendered. However, both the measures taken by the private sector and those taken by the federal and state governments could neither stem the tide of service consumption nor the escalating cost of these services to employers and taxpayers. At this juncture, employers and health insurance companies concluded that health care providers would not control the cost of service delivery. As a consequence, they decided that they must become directly involved in the clinical decisions that are also cost decisions; decisions such as, who should receive health care services, what type of services are appropriate, when and where they should be delivered, and in what quantity and for what duration they should be provided. Simply put, the employers, and the insurance companies from whom they purchased their employees' health insurance plans, decided that the only way in which they could contain costs would be for them to proactively manage the services for which they were paying, i.e., "to manage care." Thus the era of managed care in the private sector was born. It would not be until 1997 that the federal government, under ever escalating pressure to reduce the cost of taxpayer supported health care, followed suit. In that year, Congress passed Public Law No. 105-33, House Resolution 2015—the Balanced Budget Act (BBA). A portion of this act mandated that HCFA reduce Medicare expenditures by approximately $115 billion over a period of five years. To accomplish this mandate, HCFA determined that it must follow the path taken by the private sector. It recognized that it must shift the method of Medicare reimbursement from a cost-based system to a PPS. To this end, HCFA instituted a PPS for rehabilitation services provided in skilled nursing facilities on July 1, 1998,[7,8] and a PPS for outpatient rehabilitation services on January 1, 1999.[9–12] A PPS for home health care is expected to begin on October 1, 1999[13,14] and a PPS for inpatient acute rehabilitation is scheduled to be introduced on October 1, 2000. (Appendix 1–A at the end of this chapter contains a list of key managed care terms that are used frequently in this text. They explain some of the basic components of managed care systems and practices.)

MANAGED CARE: ITS GOAL, SYSTEM, AND PROCESS

What Is Managed Care?

According to Griffin,[15] managed care systems integrate the financing and delivery of health care services to members of a managed care plan by the following means:

- arrangements with select providers to furnish comprehensive health services to plan members
- explicit standards for the selection of health care providers
- formal programs of ongoing quality assurance or utilization review
- significant financial incentives for members to use providers and procedures associated with the plan

At this time, only 5 percent of employes in the United States are enrolled in unmanaged fee-for-service health plans.[16] As a consequence, the majority of providers must contract with managed care plans in order to maintain their patient volume.

What Is the Goal of Managed Care?

Managed care's goal is cost containment and quality enhancement. Quality frequently means something different to the payer than it does to the therapist. The payer views quality as the efficient use of the funds available for health care, appropriate use of health care resources, and maximum possible contribution of health care to reduction in lost productivity.[17] The payer defines quality in terms of how the therapist utilizes resources to reach a desired patient outcome and the degree to which that outcome reduces other costs associated with the problem being treated. Therapists define quality in terms such as achieving maximal functional patient independence and attaining an outcome that restores or enhances the patient's quality of life. To function effectively within the managed care environment, the therapist must incorporate the payer's definition of quality into his or her own.

What Are the Systems That Manage Health Care?

These systems, often referred to as managed care organizations (MCOs), vary widely in the degree to which they exert control over member access to and utilization of health care services. Employers most frequently use one of the following three types of plans.

Indemnity Insurance Plans

This is the traditional fee-for-service health care plan in which the insurance carrier pays 80 percent of the bill and patients pay 20 percent, as well as the amount of their deductible. This system had few methods for constraining resource utilization. In recent years, fee-for-service plans have instituted some forms of prospective and concurrent utilization review and case management. Employers are the primary clients of insurance carriers and they shop for the lowest premium. In response, the insurance carriers are moving away from this expensive type of plan and developing managed care plans.

Preferred Provider Organization (PPO)

A PPO is a group of health care providers (which may include both physicians and hospitals) that contracts with employers, insurance carriers, or the government to provide services. A PPO is paid on the basis of a discounted rate. Members of PPO plans choose either a preferred provider (a physician, hospital, or other health care entity that has contracted with the PPO plan) or a provider of their own. There are few restrictions on service utilization in this system. The member has a financial incentive to use preferred providers: when they do, their copayment and deductible are typically reduced. PPOs also employ some form of utilization review.

Health Maintenance Organization (HMO)

HMOs are organized systems that provide a defined and comprehensive set of basic and supplemental health maintenance and treatment services. They provide services for a specific geographic area and employers contract with HMOs. Private citizens and Medicare beneficiaries who reside in that area may voluntarily enroll in an HMO. They also establish a network of providers and require their members to obtain services from within that network. Some HMOs offer plans to their members that allow them to choose service providers outside of the network. These plans are more expensive, and are called point-of-service (POS) plans.

HMOs employ numerous methods to control member access and utilization of services. Each member must choose a primary care physician (PCP) from within the system. The PCP acts as a gatekeeper who controls the member's access to all services. The PCP either provides the services or seeks approval from the HMO's utilization committee to refer the member to a specialist, admit the member to a hospital for inpatient care, or to arrange for outpatient and home health rehabilitation services. HMOs also require preadmission certification and employ case management and prospective, concurrent, and retrospective review. The U.S. health care delivery system continues to evolve. The types and names of today's MCOs will undoubtedly change; however, the HMO model of service delivery and control is the foundation upon which future systems will be developed.

Managed Care's Process: How Does It Pay?

Both the private sector's and Medicare's non-HMO approach to payment is based on a PPS. However, while both use a PPS, they differ significantly in that the private sector negotiates payment rates with providers and Medicare does not.

Private Sector PPS

MCOs negotiate a set rate of payment with providers prior to the delivery of services. For inpatient rehabilitation, this rate, usually a per diem rate, covers all services provided. As such, the provider takes the risk that the agreed-upon rate of payment will be sufficient to cover all costs incurred in providing rehabilitation to a given client. If the actual cost of service provision is greater than the agreed-upon per diem rate, the provider loses money. If the cost is less than the per diem rate, the provider makes money. Outpatient rehabilitation is usually based on a negotiated reduced fee-for-service rate as well as the number of treatment visits that will be allowed. Here, the provider must again be sure that the agreed-upon rate will cover all costs of providing the service. Access to rehabilitation services is controlled by a client's primary care physician. MCO case managers monitor the effectiveness of rehabilitation once it begins and make recommendations to the PCP as to whether continued rehabilitation should be authorized. In the future, MCOs may move toward a case-rate method of payment. This payment model is based on a negotiated rate for a particular diagnostic group, such as stroke or spinal cord injury, rather than on an individual client basis. Eventually a payment model may evolve that will encompass the entire span of services. Such a model, sometimes referred to as disease state management, will be based on a rate of reimbursement that covers the entire course of care, from acute care to inpatient rehabilitation through outpatient rehabilitation.

Medicare PPS

The PPS implemented by HCFA in skilled nursing facilities on July 1, 1998, is a type of capitated payment arrangement with skilled nursing facility providers of rehabilitation and/or other medical services. Medicare's PPS differs from that of the private sector's in that it is not only based on a preset rate of reimbursement but also a specified minimum amount of service (speech-language pathology, occupational therapy, and physical therapy) that must be provided per week, the number of days the services must be provided, and the amount of time spent in each service. One component of HCFA's method of determining what it will pay for rehabilitation is based on the intensity of services required by a given client. Required intensity of service is determined in two ways. One way is that of categorizing clients into resource utilization groups (RUGs). There are seven major RUGs: Rehabilitation; Extensive Services; Special Care; Clinically Complex; Impaired Cognition; Behavior; and Reduced Physical Function. Only those clients who fall into the rehabilitation RUG qualify for rehabilitation services. The rehabilitation RUG is divided into five subcategories: Ultra High; Very High; High; Medium; and Low. Ultra High represents the most intensive level of care needs and Low represents the least intense. As shown in Figure 1–1, each category specifies a minimum amount of therapy that must be provided, the number of disciplines required to provide it, and the frequency of their interventions. A client is placed in one of these five categories on the basis of rehabilitation services that were provided during the initial assessment period. It is important to note that the type of disciplines (i.e., speech-language pathology, occupational therapy, physical therapy, and recreational therapy) are not specified. It is the responsibility of provider management and the rehabilitation team to determine the most appropriate allocation of the required therapy among these disciplines on the basis of prevailing client needs. The intensity of a client's caregiving needs is the second way of determining level of payment. As shown in Figure 1–2, each of the five

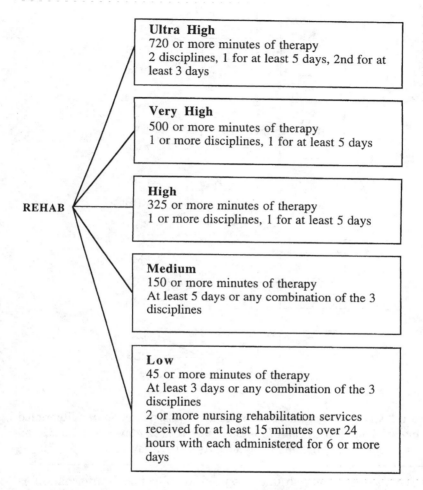

Ultra High
720 or more minutes of therapy
2 disciplines, 1 for at least 5 days, 2nd for at
least 3 days

Very High
500 or more minutes of therapy
1 or more disciplines, 1 for at least 5 days

High
325 or more minutes of therapy
1 or more disciplines, 1 for at least 5 days

REHAB

Medium
150 or more minutes of therapy
At least 5 days or any combination of the 3
disciplines

Low
45 or more minutes of therapy
At least 3 days or any combination of the 3
disciplines
2 or more nursing rehabilitation services
received for at least 15 minutes over 24
hours with each administered for 6 or more
days

Figure 1–1 Classification Based on Therapy Intensity. *Source:* Reprinted from Interim Final Rule, *Federal Register*, Vol. 63, (12 May 1998): 26252 and HCFA Implementing Program Memoranda A-98-16, (May 1998).

---

rehabilitation RUGs is divided into the three subcategories of C, B, and A; specifically, RUC (Rehab Ultra High—C), RUB (Rehab Ultra High—B), and RUA (Rehab Ultra High—A). Category C is the highest intensity of care and A is the least. The designation of C, B, or A is determined by the client's activities of daily living (ADL) score on the Minimal Data Set Version 2.0 (MDS 2.0).[18] The MDS 2.0 is a clinical assessment instrument developed by HCFA. It is used in skilled nursing facilities by therapists and nurses to identify client care needs and establish the plan of care to meet

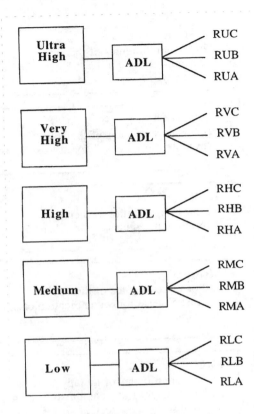

Figure 1–2 Classification Based on Intensity of Assistance. *Source:* Reprinted from Interim Final Rule, *Federal Register*, Vol. 63, (12 May 1998): 26252 and HCFA Implementing Program Memoranda A-98-16, (May 1998).

them. This assessment instrument is used to collect such information as diagnosis, medications, nursing rehabilitation needs, and ADL capabilities. It also provides the means by which the team assesses cognition, communication/hearing, vision, mood and behavior, physical functioning, and dental status. While the client is assessed in all of these areas, only the ADL scores for transfers, bed mobility, toileting, and eating (found in section G, Physical Functioning and Structural Problems, of the MDS 2.0) are used to designate a given client as either C, B, or A. The two following scales from the MDS 2.0 are used to rate a client's performance in each of these four ADL domains:

- Self-Performance Scale
  0 = independent
  1 = supervised

2 = limited assistance
3 = extensive assistance
4 = total dependence
• ADL Support Provided
0 = no setup or physical help from staff
1 = setup only
2 = one person physical assist
3 = two+ persons physical assist

Both the amount of therapy a client requires (Ultra High, Very High, High, Medium, or Low) and the required degree of ADL assistance (C, B, or A) are factored in to determine the per diem rate that HCFA will pay for a given client's rehabilitation. Using the approximate HCFA (federal) per diem rates for Ultra High, High, and Medium RUGs as an example (Figure 1–3), it can be seen that the higher the therapy intensity category and the

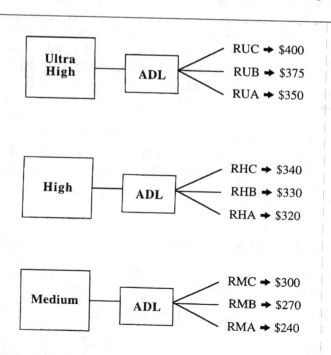

Figure 1–3 Payment Based on Intensity of Therapy and Caregiving Needs. *Source:* Reprinted from *Federal Register*, Vol. 63, No. 91, pp. 26000252–26000316, 1998. Department of Health and Human Services, Health Care Financing Administration.

greater the level of assistance required within that category, the higher will be the rate of reimbursement. These rates cover all of the costs of therapy and nursing services as well as medical supplies, medications, and laboratory studies. HCFA will adjust the rates on an annual basis.

In order to ease the fiscal impact on providers, HCFA will phase in the full federal rate over a period of four years, beginning July 1, 1998. This will be accomplished by providing a blended rate of reimbursement, which is based on a percentage of the federal rate plus a percentage of the provider's cost. During the first year, this blended per diem rate will be based on 25 percent of the federal rate and 75 percent of the provider's costs, the second year it will be based on 50 percent of the federal rate and 50 percent of the provider's cost; and, in the third year it will move to 75 percent of the federal rate and 25 percent of the provider's cost. When the fourth year is reached, the federal rate will be the sole basis for reimbursement. Using an example federal rate of $400 for the Ultra High RUG, Level C (RUC) and an example provider per diem cost of $700 for that same category of client, one can readily see (Table 1–1) that the Medicare PPS will have a significant fiscal impact on providers of rehabilitation. Even with HCFA's blended rate approach, the rate of reimbursement to a hypothetical provider whose per diem costs are $700 will start out below its current cost to provide the service and become progressively worse over the following three years. As a consequence, providers will either have to find ways to bring their costs in line with the federal rate, not provide services to Medicare beneficiaries, or go out of business. Since Medicare beneficiaries represent the largest population receiving rehabilitation services, the choice will most probably be that of either reducing expenses or going out of business.

Table 1–1 Example Federal Rate Phase-in for Rehab RUG Ultra High—C

Phase-in Year	Federal Percent of $400.00	=	Federal Amount Paid	+	Provider Percent of $700.00	Allowed Provider Costs	=	Actual per Diem Paid
1	25%	=	$100.00	+	75%	$525.00	=	$625.00
2	50%	=	$200.00	+	50%	$350.00	=	$550.00
3	75%	=	$300.00	+	25%	$175.00	=	$475.00
4	100%	=	$400.00	+	0%	$ 0.	=	$400.00

HCFA took a different approach to managing inpatient and outpatient Medicare Part B therapy services.[19-22] On January 1, 1999, it imposed both a fee schedule and dollar amount cap on speech-language pathology, physical therapy, and occupational therapy services provided in an outpatient setting. The fee schedule sets the amount that HCFA will pay for each speech-language pathology, physical therapy, and occupational therapy evaluation and treatment procedure. It is based on the American Medical Association's (AMA) Resource-Based Relative Value Scale (RBRVS).[23] The RBRVS consists of three components: (1) the work required to provide a procedure, (2) the expense of running one's clinical practice, and (3) the expense of malpractice insurance.

In the context of RBRVS, work is defined as consisting of five elements:

1. The amount of time required to provide a procedure
2. The technical skill required to provide the procedure
3. The amount of mental effort and judgment required to provide the procedure
4. The amount of psychological stress experienced providing the procedure
5. The degree of physical effort required to provide the service

These five elements are used to determine the value of one clinical procedure in relation to another, a procedure "relative value." For example, if procedure A requires twice the time, technical skill, mental effort, and judgment, and involves twice the amount of psychological stress and physical effort as procedure B, then the relative value of service A would be twice that of service B. In the RBRVS, all procedures are described as "current terminology procedures" (CPT) and assigned a number referred to as a CPT code. For example, 92506 is evaluation of speech, language, voice; 92507 is treatment of speech, language, voice, communication; 97250 is myofascial release/soft tissue mobilization, one or more regions; and 97500 is orthotics training (dynamic bracing, splinting), upper and/or lower extremities. HCFA's fee schedule for speech-language pathology, occupational therapy, and physical therapy consists of the CPT codes that describe the procedures provided by each of these disciplines and the preset dollar amount that will be paid for each. Each procedure is paid at the rate dictated by its relative value. The procedure codes for speech-language pathology, physical therapy, occupational therapy, psychology, and social work can be found in the *Physician's Current*

Procedural Terminology book.[24] This book does not, however, list the dollar amount that will be paid for each procedure.

In addition to controlling the amount paid per procedure, HCFA also placed a $1,500 cap on Part B services provided by skilled nursing facilities, home health agencies, and comprehensive outpatient rehabilitation facilities (CORFs). At this time, speech-language pathology and physical therapy share a $1,500 cap, and occupational therapy has a separate $1,500 cap. This cap was not, however, placed on rehabilitation services provided by hospital outpatient departments.Thus, HCFA not only controls the amount that will be paid for each procedure, but also limits the total amount it will pay per patient per discipline when services are provided in the settings noted above. However, at this time, these caps only apply to the total amount a single-provider can charge. A client is not prohibited from obtaining services from a second or even a third provider up to the single-provider caps. It is the responsibility of each provider to track the dollar amount of services rendered and terminate treatment when the cap for each discipline has been reached. As noted earlier, rehabilitation services provided in hospital-based outpatient departments are exempt from these caps; however, they are not exempt from HCFA's fee schedule or the possibility that the charges will be denied retrospectively if they are found to be not medically necessary. As noted earlier in this chapter, the BBA also mandates that HCFA implement a PPS for home health by October 1, 1999, and a PPS for inpatient acute rehabilitation by October 1, 2000. At this time, it is not known whether the PPSs for these levels of care will be the same as the SNF of outpatient PPSs.

CONCLUSION

The current systemwide transformation of healthcare is the result of powerful cost-cutting pressures. These pressures are moving the reimbursement of rehabilitation services from a fee-for-service and cost reimbursement method of payment to a PPS. The changes in reimbursement methods will act to alter and reshape our historical approach to the delivery of rehabilitation services. In this new health care environment, payers will expect providers to manage their costs (Exhibit 1–1) and, in turn, providers will rely on therapists to assist them in day-to-day cost management (Exhibit 1–2).

Exhibit 1–1 Payer Expectations

Payers will expect providers to manage their costs by:
- providing proof of cost-effectiveness
- providing proof of treatment effectiveness
- specifying the client's outcome before the commencement of treatment
- specifying the type, frequency, and intensity of treatment (costs) before commencement of treatment
- producing outcomes that prevent the reoccurrence of the same problem or occurrence of associated new problems
- producing durable outcomes
- creating high customer satisfaction

In essence, the therapist will be expected to provide the highest possible quality of care that results in the greatest value to all stakeholders (i.e., payer, provider, therapist, and client); doing so is not foreign to therapists. However, in the fee-for-service era of rehabilitation, quality was defined as providing whatever services the therapists felt necessary regardless of cost. Today, quality is defined as the provision of the most appropriate, effective, and efficient services (Exhibit 1–3) that result in the best outcome (Exhibit 1–4).

Exhibit 1–2 Provider Expectations

Providers will need therapists to manage costs by:
- directing treatment toward a predetermined "whole person" outcome
- achieving the projected "whole person" outcome at or below the rate of reimbursement
- managing the course of rehabilitation on the basis of critical pathways that are tied to an objectively defined and individualized "whole person" outcome
- managing the course of rehabilitation on the basis of an expected performance pathway (i.e., functional, measurable, and time-framed short-term goals that parallel the critical pathway)
- treating within the context of an interdisciplinary treatment plan
- providing treatment based on standardized treatment protocols
- using the most clinically effective treatment approaches
- using the most cost-effective treatment approaches
- producing an outcome that is durable
- creating high customer satisfaction

Exhibit 1–3 Components of Quality

Appropriate: The utilization of only those assessment and treatment procedures that are known to be the most specific to the needs of a particular diagnostic group or an individual within that group.
Effective: The utilization of only those assessment and treatment procedures that are known to have the highest correlation with the greatest functional gains for specific diagnostic group or individual within that group.
Efficient: The utilization of only those assessment and treatment procedures that are known to have the highest correlation with both the greatest functional gains and the least frequency, intensity, and duration of treatment.

Exhibit 1–4 Best Outcome

Rehabilitation services that result in:
- A client's ability to participate in life to the fullest extent possible
- No readmission to rehabilitation for the condition that was originally treated
- The prevention of complications
- Increased overall wellness
- High customer satisfaction

Exhibit 1–5 Valued Rehabilitation Outcomes

- Services that result in the highest cost/benefit ratio (i.e., the best outcome for the least cost)
- Services that result in a durable outcome (i.e., eliminate readmission to rehabilitation for the same condition caused by the original medical episode)
- Services that reduce the utilization of collateral and/or healthcare services unrelated to the original medical episode (i.e., prevention of secondary complications related to the original medical episode and/or wellness interventions for at-risk clients such as restroke and diet management of diabetic clients)
- Services that result in high customer satisfaction

In the health care environment of today, quality is assumed and value is sought. Payers, employers, and healthcare policy makers want evidence of cost-effectiveness and treatment efficacy. In the past providers of rehabilitation were challenged by the question, "does rehabilitation produce results?" The question asked today is, "do the results that you produce make a difference? (i.e., Do the results create value?)" (Exhibit 1–5).

REFERENCES

1. M. Burcham, "Managing Change," *Rehab Management* 7, no. 1 (1994): 105–106.
2. K. Griffin and M. Fazen, *Quality Improvement Digest* (winter 1993): 1–8.
3. Griffin and Fazen, *Quality Improvement Digest*, 1.
4. Griffin and Fazen, *Quality Improvement Digest*, 1.
5. L. Strasen, *Key Business Skills for Nurse Managers* (Philadelphia: J.B. Lippincott Co., 1987), 1–12.
6. S. Wolk and T. Blair, *Trends in Medical Rehabilitation* (Reston, VA: American Rehabilitation Association, 1994), 33.
7. "Interim Final Rule," *Federal Register* 63, (12 May 1998): 26252.
8. "HCFA Implementing Program Memoranda A-98-16," (May 1998).
9. "Proposed Rule," *Federal Register* 63, (5 June 1998): 30818.
10. "Final Rule," *Federal Register* 63, (2 November 1998): 58814.
11. "Proposed Rule," *Federal Register* 63, (8 September 1998): 47552.
12. "HCFA Implementing Program Memoranda A-98-8, A-98-24, and AB-98-63," (March 1998, July 1998, October 1998).
13. "Final Rule," *Federal Register* 63, (1 June 1997): 29648.
14. "Final Rule," *Federal Register* 63, (4 March 1998): 10730.
15. Griffin and Fazen, *Quality Improvement Digest*, 1.
16. P. Starr, *The Logic of Health Care Reform* (New York: Penguin USA, 1994), 1–10.
17. N. Beckley, Rehab Administration under Managed Care, *Rehab Management* 9, no. 1 (1996): 27–31.
18. *Long Term Care Facility Resident Assessment Instrument User's Manual* (Natuck, MA: Eliot Press, 1995).
19. "Proposed Rule," *Federal Register* 63, (5 June 1998): 30818.
20. "Final Rule," *Federal Register* 63, (2 November 1998): 58814.
21. "Proposed Rule," *Federal Register* 63, (8 September 1998): 47552.
22. "HCFA Implementing Program Memoranda A-98-8, A-98-24, and AB-98-63," (March 1998, July 1998, October 1998).
23. American Medical Association, *Medicare RBRVS: The Physicians Guide* (Chicago: 1999), 1–61.
24. American Medical Association, *Physicians Current Procedural Terminology*, 5th ed. (Chicago: 1999).

SUGGESTED READING

Clifton, D. 1997. Long-Term Care Therapy: Opportunities and Threats. *Rehab Management* December/January: 28.

DeJong, G. and Sutton, J. 1995. Rehab 2000: The Evolution of Medical Rehabilitation in American Health Care. In *Outcome-Oriented Rehabilitation: Principles, Strategies, and Tools for Effective Program Management*, eds. P.K. Landrum, N.D. Schmidt, and A. McLean, 3–40. Gaithersburg, MD: Aspen Publishers, Inc.

Higgins, W. 1991. Rationing Medical Care. *Family Medicine* May/June: 292–296.

Knight, W. 1998. *Managed Care: What It Is and How It Works*. Gaithersburg, MD: Aspen Publishers, Inc.

Kongstvedt, P.R. 1997. *Essentials of Managed Care*, 2d. ed. Gaithersburg, MD: Aspen Publishers, Inc.

Rao, P. and Freda, M. 1995. Rehab's Sea of Change. *Rehab Management 8*, no. 6: 62–67.

Rausch, R. 1995. Succeeding under Capitation. *Rehab Management 8,* no. 4: 135–136.

Rognehaugh, R. 1998. *The Managed Health Care Dictionary*, 2d ed. Gaithersburg, MD: Aspen Publishers, Inc.

Shi, L. and Singh, D.A. 1998. *Delivering Health Care in America: A System Approach*. Gaithersburg, MD: Aspen Publishers, Inc.

Zimmerman, D. and Skalko, J. 1994. *Reengineering Health Care: A Vision for the Future*. Franklin, WI: Eagle Press.

Appendix 1-A
Understanding the Language:
Key Managed Care Terms

- **Authorization:** Approval of health care services, such as rehabilitation, before the service is rendered.
- **Capitation:** A method of payment to providers. Capitated payment is a fixed amount of money set by contract between the managed care plan and the provider. The provider is paid this amount of money regardless of the type and amount of services required or the costs incurred to render them.
- **Case Management:** A system of monitoring and coordinating a member's course of treatment, particularly those cases that involve high cost or extensive services. Case management may involve assessment, treatment planning, service coordination, progress monitoring, and managing the member's total care to ensure optimal outcomes.
- **Case Manager:** An individual employed by a managed care plan (external case manager) and an individual employed by the provider (internal case manager) to carry out the case management process. The majority of case managers are nurses.
- **Copayment:** A fixed amount that the member must pay to the provider at the time service is rendered.
- **Discounted Fee For Service:** A method of payment in which the managed care plan pays a fixed percentage of the provider's full charges (e.g., 80 percent of charges).
- **Fee For Service:** A method of payment in which the provider is paid the full amount of billed charges for services rendered. This payment method does not occur in a managed care plan.
- **Enrollee:** Same as member.
- **Gatekeeper:** An individual who controls a member's access to and use of health care services. The member's PCP is usually the gatekeeper.

Source: Reprinted from R. Rognehaugh, *The Managed Health Care Dictionary*, 2d. Ed., © 1998, Aspen Publishers, Inc.

- **Independent Practice Association (IPA):** An IPA is comprised of physicians in separate private practices who contract with managed care organizations (MCOs) to provide services to the MCOs' members, either on a capitated or reduced fee-for-service basis. An IPA includes both generalists and specialists.
- **Member:** An individual who has enrolled in a managed care plan and any eligible dependent.
- **Per Diem Rate:** A form of capitation. It is a fixed amount, usually for all services that will be required, that a managed care plan pays for a day regardless of the amount and cost of rehabilitation services required to reach a projected outcome.
- **Preadmisson Certification:** The determination that a member needs hospitalization and the estimated length of stay in the hospital before admission.
- **Primary Care:** Medical services provided by internists, family practitioners, obstetricians, gynecologists, and/or pediatricians in an ambulatory or inpatient setting.
- **Primary Care Physician (PCP):** A physician who provides primary care services. The PCP has the responsibility for a member's overall course of treatment and determines whether the member requires more costly services, such as medical specialists, rehabilitation, and/or hospitalization. Each member of a managed care plan selects his or her PCP from a list of physicians provided by the plan.
- **Provider:** A person, entity, or facility that provides medical care or services.
- **Risk Pool:** An MCO withholds a portion of the money it has agreed to pay a provider for services rendered and uses this money to create financial reserves. These financial reserves—risk pool—are used to pay for unanticipated utilization of services. If funds are left over at the end of a specified period of time (usually a year), they are split between the MCO and the provider. The funds are divided based on the degree to which external services (services provided outside of the MCO) were utilized. For example, as the amount of external utilization increases, the amount of the funds paid to the provider from the risk pool decreases. Thus, the MCO uses the risk pool to encourage the provider to control referrals to specialists and/or speciality services, such as rehabilitation.

- **Shared Risk:** When services are provided on the basis of a capitated payment system or a discounted fee-for-service arrangement, the provider shares the financial risk with the managed care plan. That is, providers are at risk of not making a profit if they do not manage their costs. If the cost of care exceeds the contracted capitated rate or discounted fee, the provider must absorb the excess costs which, in turn, reduces the provider's profit.

- **Utilization Management (UM):** A systematic overall process of controlling a member's access to and utilization of medical services. It is the key tool that managed care plans use to control costs of services provided to plan members. UM includes an array of techniques, such as preadmission certification (prospective review), concurrent review, case management, hospital discharge planning, retrospective chart review, and provider profiling (i.e., evaluating the quality and efficiency of services rendered by a provider to determine whether that provider's services will continue to be used).

- **Utilization Review (UR):** A review of the appropriateness, quality, and need for services provided to plan members. UR may be *prospective* (e.g., a proposed plan of care or a discharge plan is reviewed and approved before implementation), *concurrent* (e.g., monitoring treatment procedures and patient progress during the course of rehabilitation), or *retrospective* (e.g., audits of selected medical charts after services have been provided to determine the appropriatness and quality of services rendered).

CHAPTER 2

The Business of Rehabilitation: Where Does All the Money Go?

KEY POINTS

- Rehabilitation is a business.

- Profit is not a dirty word.

- Therapists must understand basic business practice concepts.

- Therapists must understand factors critical to maintaining the fiscal health of a rehabilitation program.

- Shifts in revenue sources determine business profitability.

Rehabilitation has always been a business. Therapists, however, usually do not concern themselves with the financial side of their clinical practice. In fact, they typically view money as the concern of administration and the provision of therapy as their only concern. Therapists are trained to be devoted, caring people with knowledge and skills that are given freely to their clients. Financial issues such as a business's need to maintain a healthy profit margin are rarely, if ever, part of a therapist's clinical training. As a result, business issues such as the cost of therapy services or an employer's profit and loss status are seen as the domain of management. To carry out their clinical case manager's role and responsibilities, however, therapists must have a basic awareness, understanding, and acceptance of the business side of rehabilitation. Rehabilitation programs whose therapists do not have this understanding and expertise are in danger of extinction.

PROFIT IS NOT A DIRTY WORD

The basis of any business is the sale of a product to a consumer for a price that provides the business owner with a profit. In the business of rehabilitation, the product is service and therapy is the type of service. Services are obtained and provided through a food chain (see Figure 2–1) in which money is the food.

There are two consumers of rehabilitation services: (1) the entity that pays for them (e.g., employers, governmental programs, and clients who have paid for a portion of their health care plan via copayments) and (2) the client who receives the services. The therapists' employer (hereafter referred to as the "provider") sells therapy services to these consumers for a price that will return a profit. The provider pays therapists to provide the services to the consumer. The therapist provides the services and the provider bills the consumer (hereafter referred to as the "payer") for them at the agreed-upon price. The money the provider receives is used, in part to pay for therapist's work, as well as all other expenses (costs) that were incurred in the provision of service. Thus the "food chain" is completed. In a very basic sense, the business side of rehabilitation operates no differently than the way in which an average working individual manages his or her personal finances. Workers sell their knowledge and skills (a product) to an employer in order to generate revenue (paycheck), which they use to purchase goods and services and pay bills (costs). They strive to control costs so that some money will be left after bills are paid (profit). They invest some of their profit into savings (financial reserves) and use the remainder for discretionary spending. Managing costs in order to make a profit is as key to managing one's personal finances as it is to running a profitable rehabilitation business.

Whether you work in a for-profit or not-for-profit setting, the business goal is the same: to make a profit. There is no such thing as a "nonprofit organization." Both types of businesses must make a profit in order to survive. The difference between the two relates to the manner in which profits are used. The for-profit rehabilitation business uses its profits to improve and expand services, build financial reserves (a savings account that is used to pay for unforeseen expenses), *and* to distribute a portion of the profits to the shareholders and/or the owner. In a not-for-profit rehabilitation business, the profits are only used to improve and expand services

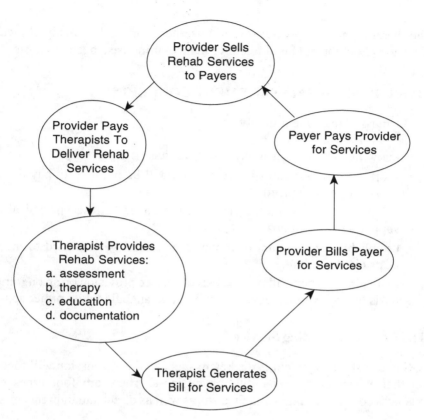

Figure 2–1 Rehabilitation Food Chain

---

and build financial reserves. Neither type of business can operate for very long if it regularly spends more than it receives in income.

A Business Cannot Spend More Than It Earns

In the current health care economy, a rehabilitation business can no longer make a profit by raising the price (charges) of the service or by increasing the number of clients treated (volume). Not only have payers decreased the amount they are willing to pay for these services, but they also are tightly controlling lengths of stay and levels of care. In this era of rehabilitation, profitability will be realized through cost management and the therapist plays a pivotal role in this endeavor. Today, many clinical decisions hold the potential to either reduce or increase business costs.

BASIC BUSINESS MANAGEMENT CONCEPTS

Business management involves:

- knowing what it costs to provide a service
- projecting the amount of revenue that will be required to pay these costs and make a profit
- setting a price for the service that the payer will accept and also supports the profit goal
- establishing the amount of money that cannot be exceeded to meet costs (setting a budget)
- managing and controlling the costs of service provision on an ongoing basis to stay within weekly, monthly, and annual budget projections

The Costs of Providing Service

Since cost management is the key to success, this discussion will focus on that aspect of the rehabilitation business. There are four types of business costs: fixed and variable costs as well as direct and indirect costs.

Fixed and Variable Costs

Fixed costs are those expenses that remain at the same fixed level regardless of the number of clients treated. Whether a therapist treats one or eight clients a day, these costs remain the same.[1] Exhibit 2–1 shows an example of fixed costs.

Variable costs are those that either increase or decrease as the number of clients treated increases or decreases.[2] (See Exhibit 2–2.)

The total cost of running a rehabilitation business is the sum of the fixed and variable costs. (See Exhibit 2–3.)

Direct and Indirect Costs

Certain types of labor (personnel), materials, and equipment are required to provide the therapy and certain types of labor, materials, and

Exhibit 2–1 Example of Fixed Costs

Monthly salaries for a 15-bed rehabilitation unit:	
Therapists	$ 36,000.00
Nurses	23,000.00
Administration	24,000.00
(Medical records dept.)	
Housekeeping dept.	6,600.00
Maintenance dept.	3,400.00
Plant operations	15,716.00
Building/Fixtures	5,000.00
Equipment	1,200.00
Other administration	8,000.00
Human resources dept., Billing dept., Loan payments	
Total monthly fixed costs:	$ 122,916.00
Total annual fixed costs:	$1,474,992.00

equipment are required for their support. Of the fixed and variable costs listed above, some are generated during the actual provision of therapy and, consequently, are called *direct costs*. On the other hand, some of these fixed and variable costs are created by the support systems that are required to provide the therapy. These are called *indirect costs*. Direct and indirect costs are not different from fixed and variable costs; rather they are categories into which fixed and variable costs are placed.[3] (See Exhibit 2–4.) Why should this seemingly arcane bit of information be of interest to rehabilitation therapists? For two reasons: (1) If the volume of clients

---

Exhibit 2–2 Example of Variable Costs

Costs per patient, per patient day for a 15-bed rehabilitation unit:	
Medical records	$ 29.00
Expendable therapy material	.50
Laundry and linen	5.00
Medical supplies	17.00
Expendable supplies used by the departments listed above	.50
Patient food	19.00
Total daily variable costs per client	$ 71.00
Total monthly variable costs for 15 clients:	$ 31,950.00
Total annual variable costs for 15 clients:	$383,400.00

Exhibit 2–3 Example of Total Costs

Example of total costs for a 15-bed rehabilitation unit:	
Fixed costs (monthly)	$ 122,916.00
Variable costs (monthly)	31,950.00
Total costs per month	$ 154,866.00
Total annual costs	$1,858,392.00

treated or the amount that is paid for treatment decreases, the direct costs for providing service must also be immediately decreased or (2) if the amount that is paid for treatment decreases, the direct cost for providing service must be immediately reduced as well. This process will have an impact on therapists and involve them directly in its solution.

Using the previous examples of fixed and variable costs, one can readily see that labor (salaries) comprises the greatest direct and indirect cost; yet it is also the cost that is the most controllable. If client volume decreases, so must labor costs, unless the price of service goes up, which is very unlikely. If prices decrease, then labor costs must also decrease; otherwise volume must increase without increasing costs (i.e., therapists must do more and do it more efficiently).

Projecting the Cost per Unit of Service

To realize a profit from the provision of therapy, the price charged for it must be higher than the cost of providing it. To set the price appropriately, the provider must know what it costs to provide one unit of that service.

Exhibit 2–4 Direct and Indirect Costs

Example of direct costs:	Example of indirect costs:
Therapists' salaries and benefits	Administration
Therapy supplies	Nursing
Therapy equipment	Medical records
	Housekeeping
	Laundry and linen
	Maintenance
	Utilities
	Loans

Depending upon the setting in which a therapist practices, a unit of service (UOS) is measured differently. In inpatient rehabilitation, the UOS is a *patient day* (a period of 24 hours); a UOS in outpatient rehabilitation is usually 15 minutes or some fraction of an hour; and in the home health setting the UOS is a *visit*. To determine the cost of a physical therapy (PT), occupational therapy (OT), or speech-language pathology (SLP) UOS, both the direct and indirect costs associated with that UOS must be identified. The direct UOS costs are determined by dividing the total direct costs generated by each therapy department (cost center) during a specified period of time by the total UOS provided by it during the same period of time. A year is usually the period of time used for this calculation.

The amount of the indirect costs of providing a UOS are determined by allocating a percentage of the provider's total indirect cost to each cost center. The allocation of these costs is based on specific criteria that are intended to distribute these costs fairly among the various cost centers on the basis of the amount of the support services each utilizes. For example, the percentage of the cost of the human resources and medical records departments may be allocated to a given cost center on the basis of the number of employees in that department. The reasoning here is that the larger the department, the greater will be its utilization of support services. On the other hand, the cost of the maintenance and housekeeping departments may be allocated on the basis of the total square footage a cost center requires to provide its service. The greater amount of space used by a given department, the greater will be the proportion of costs of maintenance and housekeeping allocated to that department.

Setting the Price of Service

Historically, the provider of the service has always set the price—or the fee—for a UOS. The price was typically determined by three factors: (1) the provider's profit margin goal, (2) what the payer was willing to pay, and (3) the competition. The provider's profit margin goal, then, was a set amount of money above the business's break-even point. This scenario is not always the case today, however. In many instances, it is the payer who sets the price. Many health insurance plans only allow their members to receive services from providers that have agreed to discount their fees to a certain level that is set by the insurance company. Managed care organizations (MCOs) contract with providers on the basis of capitated rates—a dollar amount that is agreed upon before the service is delivered and which is the amount paid regardless of the eventual cost of the service. This shift from provider to payer price setting coincidentally has shifted the provider's role from simply generating revenue to controlling costs.

Total Gross and Net Revenue Defined

Total gross revenue is the amount of money a provider has at the end of any given month prior to paying for business costs. *Net revenue* is the amount of money remaining after the provider has paid all business costs including those described earlier, as well as the cost of bad debts (bills for services that were never paid), denial of Medicare claims, and disallowance of charges for services that were provided.

Establishing a Budget

Managing Costs

As discussed earlier, simply breaking even is not sufficient to sustain either a for-profit or a not-for-profit rehabilitation business. Both must strive to produce a target profit margin. A rehabilitation business, like any other business, must function on the basis of a budget. Each year management must forecast expected revenue and expenses for the coming year and develop a budget that is designed to keep expenses at the level required to meet the target profit margin. Management bases its forecast on the business's previous years' known revenue and expenses, the expected increases in expenses due to natural increases in the cost of goods and services they must purchase to provide rehabilitation services, and strategies to increase their share of the rehabilitation market. In a very basic sense, then, a budget is composed of projected revenue and expenses. In general, a budget is composed of five elements: projected gross revenue, projected deductions from gross revenue, expected net gross revenue, projected expenses, and expected net income. In the sample budget (Exhibit 2–5), gross revenue is divided into that which is expected to be generated by routine services (e.g., nursing) and that which is expected to be generated by ancillary services (e.g., physical therapy, speech-language pathology, occupational therapy, and respiratory therapy). These two sources, combined, form the total gross revenue the business expects in the

Exhibit 2–5 Sample Budget

Gross Patient Revenues	
Routine patient services	$12,000,000
Ancillary services	25,000,000
Total Gross Patient Revenues	$37,000,000
Deductions from Revenues	
Provision for bad debt	$700,000
Charitable allowance	150,000
Contractual allowance	4,600,000
Total Deductions	$ 5,450,000
Net Revenues from Patients	$31,550,000
Operating Expenses	
Salaries	$14,500,000
Employee benefits	1,200,000
Medical supplies	2,500,000
Nonmedical supplies	1,400,000
Medical fees and commissions	2,200,000
Purchased services	900,000
Maintenance and utilities	1,500,000
Professional liability	350,000
Financing costs	1,200,000
Depreciation	900,000
Total Operating Expenses	$26,650,000
Net Income from Operations	$ 4,900,000
PROFIT MARGIN	15.5%

coming year. This, however, does not represent the complete revenue picture; it does not forecast the expected net gross revenue. The net gross revenue is derived by subtracting the projected dollar amount of bills that will not be paid by payers (bad debt), charges that the provider voluntarily reduces because of a client's financial hardship (charitable allowance), and negotiated rates with MCOs (contractual allowance). Next, management must project the cost (operating expenses) of providing the services that will generate the net gross revenue. The cost of service provision is then subtracted from the net gross revenue to derive the expected year-end profit (net income). The amount of the net profit dictates the provider's profit margin (the percentage the net profit is of the net gross revenue). The projected gross revenue, net gross revenue, operating expenses, and net income and expected profit margin comprise management's "operating budget." It is used on a daily, weekly, and/or monthly basis to monitor and manage the expected revenue and expenses of each revenue-producing department and the expenses of all non–revenue-producing departments. The profit margin figure is management's steering mechanism. The moment it sinks below expectations, management must quickly analyze their actual gross revenue and operating expenses to determine the source of the negative variation and take action to steer the business back on course. For example, if net gross revenue is below projections, they must either increase gross revenues, decrease deductions from revenue, or decrease expenses. If net gross revenue is on target but net income is below expectations, they must either reduce their operating expenses or increase net gross revenue. Since an operating budget is built on the expected performance of each department, management is able to identify and rectify the source of any variation from budget projections at the department level. The department manager, in turn, is responsible for monitoring the revenue and expenses of her or his department and make appropriate adjustments to maintain the department's profit margin. To achieve the desired profit margin, each cost center (therapy department) must meet or be below its budgeted costs as well as meet or exceed its budgeted UOS (revenue).

The Break-Even Point

To manage costs, one must know the business's break-even point: the point at which it neither makes nor loses money.[4] In a rehabilitation business, the break-even point is the production of the number of UOS (i.e., revenue) that is equal to the budgeted costs. Every UOS above the break-even point results in a potential profit and every UOS below it results in a potential business loss. This reality is depicted in Figure 2–2, which is based on a 15-bed inpatient rehabilitation unit. In this scenario, a UOS is a patient (client) day. The program's break-even point is a census of 8 clients per day; a census of 14 clients a day is the target profit margin. Thus, the rehabilitation program makes an increasing amount of profit as the UOS (volume of business) moves from the break-even point toward its capacity of 15 clients per day. This occurs because every UOS above the break-even point generates revenue that is not needed to pay for the program's fixed costs. While variable costs will increase with increased UOS, they will not

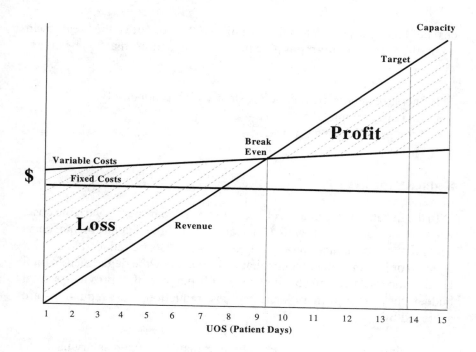

Figure 2–2 The Break-Even Point

decrease the profit margin if they have been appropriately included in the calculation of the cost of a UOS. Just as an increase in UOS above the break-even point produces a profit, a decrease below this point will produce a loss.[5] Every UOS below the break-even point is revenue that is increasingly below the program's fixed costs. While the variable costs will also decrease with a decline in UOS, such a decrease is not sufficient to offset the effect of the program's fixed costs.

MAINTAINING THE FISCAL HEALTH OF A REHABILITATION PROGRAM

Two factors are critical to a business's position relative to its break-even point: (1) fluctuations in client volume, and (2) the level of reimbursement (i.e., price). If either the volume of service or level of payment declines, the cost per UOS goes up. When the cost of a UOS rises above the break-even point, there are only four[6] possible management actions that can be taken:

1. Reduce expenses.
2. Increase and/or maintain consistently high productivity.
3. Increase volume.
4. Stop providing the service.

Reduce Expenses

In the instance of decreased client volume, a department's variable costs will naturally decrease as well. Consequently, the fixed departmental costs become the cost reduction target. Fixed costs musts be reduced to a point equal to or less than the revenue that is produced by the department's total UOS. Since salaries are 50 percent to 60 percent of a provider's total budget, they are a primary source of cost reduction. Cost reductions are achieved by

1. paying therapists on an hourly rather than on a fixed salary basis
2. using per diem therapists
3. eliminating positions
4. employing less expensive personnel to provide services

By paying staff on an hourly basis, they can be "flexed out"—sent home without pay for hours not worked that day when client volume is low. This allows the cost of therapist wages to fluctuate with the rise and fall of client volume. When therapists are paid on an hourly basis, a major portion of their costs are moved from the category of fixed expenses to that of variable expenses. The cost of employee benefits remains fixed, however.

Thus, one key to controlling the costs of therapist's wages is to have available only that number of therapists required to meet the projected demand for services (projected UOS) at any given point in time and flexing them out if and when volume dips below the projected break-even point. Per diem therapists (those paid by the day without benefits) are typically utilized when client volume rises above a level at which the budgeted staff can serve. From a cost containment perspective, however, per diem therapists should only be used for very brief periods of time since they are usually paid at a much higher rate.

The elimination of positions is another cost containment option. This is usually achieved through the consolidation of jobs. For example, the department director positions for each therapy discipline are changed to a "lead therapist" position and a single "therapy supervisor" position is created. The lead therapist is paid less than he or she was as a department director and is now responsible for producing UOS as well as for carrying some management responsibilities. The therapy supervisor is responsible for the majority of the job duties of the previous three department directors and also may be responsible for producing UOS. This approach to managing costs can also be applied to administrative positions. If the produced UOS chronically falls below the break-even point, therapist positions must be eliminated.

The utilization of less expensive personnel to deliver therapy services is yet another way of reducing the cost of wages. While PT, OT, and SLP aides are already employed to a certain degree in some rehabilitation settings, their utilization, of necessity, must and will increase in the future. The use of rehabilitation aides, however, must be based on sound clinical criteria and guidelines to ensure that the highest quality of care is preserved and the ethical responsibilities of the therapists are not violated. This can be accomplished by identifying the difference between skilled and nonskilled services. (See Chapter 3.) Costs can also be reduced by postponing budgeted expenses such as new positions, equipment, facility improvement, new programs, and/or program expansion.

Increase Productivity

There is a threshold beyond which fixed costs cannot be reduced. This is the point at which there is insufficient staff, facilities, and equipment to safely provide high-quality services. Consequently, reducing costs is only one part of the solution to managing and controlling costs; increasing the level and consistency of productivity is the other part. The higher the productivity, the lower the cost per UOS. If client volume is at the predicted level and departmental productivity is below the expected level, then action must be taken to discover the causes of this discrepancy. Action must also be taken when client volume is consistently at the predicted level and departmental productivity is only inconsistently at the expected level. In most instances, however, solving the productivity problem requires finding better ways of meeting a provider's productivity standard. To make a profit today, most providers require between six and seven productive (i.e., billable) therapy hours per day from each therapist. Productivity standards vary across the United States and sometimes across different locations within a state. The challenge, then, becomes how to meet the provider's productivity standard and accomplish all the other tasks the therapist must do, such as documentation, client conferences, team meetings, and telephone calls to physicians. From a management perspective, increasing productivity demands above the expected level for a long period of time is not cost-effective in the long run. While staff should and will rise to such occasions when they occur randomly and for short periods of time, they will rapidly feel devalued and become burned out if such productivity demands become chronic. A sense of being devalued and burned out leads to lower quality of care and high staff turnover, both of which are costly to the provider. Thus, the long-term solution to increasing productivity of existing staff is not found in simply increasing the UOS they must produce, but is found in reengineering how the work is done. (See Chapters 3, 5, 6, and 7.)

Increase Volume

Another action that can be taken when the cost of UOS rises above the break-even point is to increase the number of clients treated. Since the majority of payers do not pay the same amount that is charged for a service, however, this may not always be a viable solution. For example, Medicaid typically pays at or below a provider's break-even point. If the number of Medicaid clients served is increased, the cost per UOS will only increase. Similarly, if the provider increases the number of clients from insurance companies with which it has contracted to provide the services at a discounted rate, then the problem is also increased. Increasing volume is a viable solution only when the increased volume consists of those who pay at or near what the provider charges. Thus, the provider's "payer mix" has a strong impact on its financial stability. An optimum payer mix is one in which those who pay at or near the assessed fees outnumber those who do not. This type of payer mix is increasingly harder to achieve and will become even harder in the future. This is precisely why the provider and the provider's therapists must focus on cost management to achieve profitability.

Stop Providing the Service

This is the least attractive method of cost containment; however, if costs remain chronically higher than the break-even point, both for-profit and not-for-profit rehabilitation businesses must take this step. This could mean eliminating a particular program or completely closing the business. Just as there is a point at which one could no longer work without pay, there is also a point at which a business cannot continue without profit.

SHIFTS IN REVENUE SOURCES AFFECT BUSINESS PROFITABILITY

On the opposite side of the cost column in the business ledger is the revenue column. When a therapist renders a service, the provider bills the party responsible for paying for that service. The payer, in turn, pays for services rendered. This payment is the provider's source of revenue. Typical sources of revenue are:

* the federal Medicare program
* state Medicaid programs
* indemnity insurance plans
* managed care organizations
* individual private payment (copays or full pay)

Medicare

As noted in Chapter 1, the Medicare program is moving away from a cost and/or reasonable charges method of reimbursement to a prospective payment system (PPS). This will occur between July 1, 1998, and sometime in the year 2000 or 2001. Further, as discussed in Chapter 1, this shift in method of payment will have a significant negative impact on the profitability of providers. The effect of Medicare's implementation of a PPS is compounded by the fact that the provider, increasingly, can no longer shift costs to the private payer. That is, as more and more employers contract with MCOs, providers will not be able to make up the decreased revenue from Medicare by increasing the amount charged to private payers.

Medicaid

Medicaid employs two cost control systems: (1) prior authorization and (2) a fee schedule. The provider must submit a request for the service, called a treatment authorization request (TAR), before providing any service. The TAR contains the type of service requested (PT, OT, and/or SLP) and its proposed frequency and intensity (hour or half-hour).

A medical consultant reviews the TAR and either approves it as requested, approves it at a less frequent and/or intense level, or denies it. Medicaid will only approve a 30-day maximum treatment period, at the end of which a new TAR must be submitted requesting continued treatment. Medicaid pays for the approved services based on a fixed rate per evaluation and treatment procedure, which is called the schedule of maximum allowances. In most cases, this rate is either at or below the provider's cost of delivering the service.

Indemnity Insurance Plans

Indemnity insurance is the traditional fee-for-service type of health care coverage. Under such health care coverage, the insurance company agrees to compensate (indemnify) the customer for his or her medical expenses. In this payment system, the patient pays the provider for services and submits the provider's bill to the insurance company, which, in turn, reimburses the patient for the amount that he or she paid the provider. Thus, providers are paid the full amount of their charges when they treat a patient who has indemnity insurance. In a very short period of time, this method of payment will be completely replaced by managed care plans.

Managed Care Organizations

MCOs have numerous payment systems. They may pay on the basis of a negotiated discounted per person hourly rate, per diem, or a case rate. A case rate arrangement is one in which the provider has agreed to provide all services for a particular diagnostic category (i.e., case) for a specified dollar amount. The case rate could be a daily, weekly, or monthly rate or one for the entire course of rehabilitation. In a capitated rate arrangement, the MCO pays the contracting provider a fixed amount per month for each person enrolled in the MCO (per member per month fee). Then, whenever a member requires rehabilitation, the provider renders the service regardless of how much therapy is required or how many members require it at any given time.

Individual Private Payment

In a few instances, a client may not have health insurance and, therefore, pay for services out of their own financial resources. Two other, and quite frequent, sources of private pay are the annual deductible and a copay. Many health insurance plans require the client to pay a certain amount a year from their financial resources (annual deductible) before their insurance plan will cover health care services. Other plans require the client to pay a percentage (copay) of the charges for each health care service as they occur throughout a year, and some plans require both an annual deductible and a copay.

As can be seen, with the exception of indemnity insurance and outpatient Medicare services, there is a difference between what is charged for a service and what is paid for it. This has a major impact on a provider's ability to maintain the business above the break-even point, let alone to achieve its profit margin goal. The greater the number of clients treated whose rate of payment is at or near the amount that is charged, the easier it is to make a profit. Conversely, it becomes increasingly difficult to make a profit, let alone break even, as the volume of clients whose level of payment is at or below charges increases. As more clients enter rehabilitation through an MCO, the volume of those who pay close to actual charges will significantly decrease and may eventually disappear. Cost management, then, is the key to success in a managed care environment. To make a profit, providers must maintain their costs below the reimbursement rate they have negotiated with the MCO and below Medicare's payment caps. To do this, providers must know what is the actual cost of providing rehabilitation services. For example, they must know the true cost of providing a speech-language pathology, occupational therapy, or physical therapy UOS, which is usually a 15-minute block of hands on treatment time. Further, they must know the cost of producing an outcome for different diagnostic groups and within diagnostic group. For example, the cost of treating a spinal cord injury client versus a stroke versus a person with traumatic brain injury as well as the cost of treating a high quadriplegic versus a paraplegic or right hemisphere stroke versus a left hemisphere stroke. At this time, many providers do not possess this information. Information at this level of resolution was not necessary to successfully manage the business in the past. Previously, Medicare reimbursement was based on provider costs as reflected in their year-end Medicare cost report. The information required in this report was at the broad institutional and department levels. Identification and allocation of costs at this level does not have a direct relation to the actual resources consumed in the treatment of a client. Private payers reimbursed providers on the basis of their reasonable and customary charges. Again, what was charged did not have a direct relation to the actual cost of service delivery.

Now that providers must manage their costs, they must know their actual cost of service delivery. To do so, they will most likely turn to a cost analysis system such as activity based costing,[7,8] which analyzes and describes all work activities related to the production of a specific product.

According to Brimson, activity based costing has three components: (1) activity analysis—the identification of all activities involved in production of a product, (2) cost driver analysis—the determination of the cost of all activities required to produce a product in terms of its required quality and the time needed to achieve that level of quality, and (3) performance analysis—the determination of objective performance measures.[9] In rehabilitation, the product is the outcome. For example, the product of rehabilitation services (activities) provided to a client with a moderate aphasia and right upper and lower extremity hemiplegia following a left hemisphere stroke is an outcome of modified independent in personal, household, community, and leisure activities of daily living. The question then is, what does it cost to produce this outcome (i.e., product)? To determine this, all rehabilitation activities required to produce that outcome must be identified and analyzed. Using Baker's description of work analysis,[10] the following would be asked and answered:

- What rehabilitation services are absolutely needed to produce the outcome of modified independent in personal, household, community, and leisure activities of daily living?
- What amount (e.g., units of service or visits) of each of the necessary services are absolutely required to produce that outcome?
- How must each of the services be provided (e.g., individual therapy, group therapy, therapy provided by an assistant) to produce the outcome?

- How much time is required to provide each service in order to achieve the outcome?
- what does it cost to provide each necessary service for the time required to produce that outcome (i.e., quality of product)?

The process of activity based costing identifies the true total direct cost of providing the rehabilitation services that are required to produce a given outcome. To this figure is added the appropriate portion of traditional institutional overhead (indirect costs required to support the production of the outcome) costs in order to identify the total actual cost of producing an outcome. The information generated by activity based costing not only identifies the cost of producing an outcome, it also identifies therapist performance measures that become the means by which they can objectively manage costs. The three key performance measures are quality, time, and cost.[11] That is, the team will be expected to produce a particular quality outcome (level of independence in personal, household, community, work/school, and leisure activities of daily living) within a specified length of time for a specified cost. Performance measures provide management and a rehabilitation department with the means by which to make real-time clinical/cost management decisions. Performance measures can also be used to audit performance over longer periods of time for the purpose of continuous quality and cost improvement. They can be used to measure the effectiveness of the rehabilitation team or department with respect to three key business variables: (1) operations—how efficiently and effectively the team or department performs its function; (2) financial—how successful the team or department is in terms of meeting cost standards, generating revenue, and conformance to budget; and (3) marketing—to what extent is the team or department satisfying its public (i.e., clients, other team members/departments, and physicians).[12]

CONCLUSION

Providers of rehabilitation, like any other business, must make a profit to survive. During the era of fee-for-service and cost reimbursement, provider profitability was attained by rendering as much service as possible and/or generating high costs for service delivery. In a managed care system, provider profitability can only be realized through cost containment. When functioning within a PPS, profit can only be found by achieving the best possible rehabilitation outcome either at or, even better, below the cap.

During the early phase of managed care, prior to the implementation of a PPS for rehabilitation, the payers managed their costs by becoming directly involved in managing the type, frequency, and duration of services rendered to a given client. During this time period, rehabilitation services could not be provided without prior authorization. The payers' case managers authorized the type, frequency, and duration of treatment and monitored its effectiveness during the course of rehabilitation. As we move into a PPS for rehabilitation, we will experience a 180-degree turn around. When functioning under a PPS, the provider is at a financial risk. The provider will experience a financial loss if the cost of service exceeds the cap. As a consequence, the provider, of necessity, will turn to the rehabilitation team to play a major role in cost management. This is a logical move since the team's clinical decisions regarding the type, frequency, and duration of services are also cost decisions. The rehabilitation team has always been responsible for managing treatment effectiveness, now it also is responsible for managing five clinical cost drivers: (1) amount of clinical resource utilization (i.e., which disciplines should treat a given client and their frequency and intensity of intervention); (2) service delivery format (i.e., individual and group treatment, cotreatment, and aide-provided services); (3) duration of treatment; (4) the appropriate level of care; and (5) risk of complications.

REFERENCES

1. R. Hilton, *Managerial Accounting* (New York: McGraw-Hill, Inc., 1991), 26.

2. Hilton, *Managerial Accounting*, 26.

3. Hilton, *Managerial Accounting*, 26.

4. Hilton, *Managerial Accounting*, 26.

5. L. Strassen, *Key Business Skills for Nurse Managers* (Philadelphia: J.B. Lippincott Co., 1987), 97.

6. Strassen, *Key Business Skills for Nurse Managers*, 102.

7. J. Baker, *Activity-Based Costing Management and Activity-Based Management for Health Care* (Gaithersburg, MD: Aspen Publishers, Inc., 1998), 29.

8. J. Brimson and J. Antos, *Activity-Based Management for Service Industries: Government Entities and Non-Profit Organizations* (New York: John Wiley & Sons, 1994), 15–25.

9. Brimson and Antos, *Activity-Based Management for Service Industries*, 15–25.

10. Baker, *Activity-Based Costing Management and Activity-Based Management for Health Care*, 29.

11. Baker, *Activity-Based Costing Management and Activity-Based Management for Health Care*, 113.

12. R. Scott-MacStravic, "Performance Auditing for Health Care Supervisors," in *The Health Care Supervisor*, ed. C. McConnell (Gaithersburg, MD: Aspen Publishers, Inc., 1993), 13–24.

CHAPTER 3

Clinical Case Management: The Expanded Role of the Therapist

KEY POINTS

- Quality and cost management are not mutually exclusive endeavors.

- Therapists are responsible for managing both the quality and the cost of their services.

- Clinical case management is the process of producing the best possible client outcomes for the least cost.

The era of managed care brings with it a requisite change in therapists' views and understanding of their role. Therapists are now clinical case managers. They must be able to provide competent clinical care while managing and supervising resources, controlling costs, and effecting a meaningful outcome.[1] Central to success in this new role is an understanding of the shift that has occurred in the payers' definition of "quality of care." In the past, quality was defined solely as rehabilitation services that resulted in the client's attainment of the highest possible level of functional independence, regardless of the resources required to achieve it. Today, payers define quality as those rehabilitation services that are both effective and efficient.

Effective services are those that result in:

- the attainment of skills and abilities that are meaningful and useful in the client's natural environment,

- the retention of these skills and abilities across time without the need for further intervention, and
- the reduction or prevention of risk for future complications that would require further health care services.

Efficient services are those that attain the best possible client outcome at the least possible cost.

The new definition of quality retains the focus on functional independence but adds three new dimensions: (1) outcome durability, (2) prevention of rehospitalization, and (3) cost of care. This new definition indicates that while it is the therapists' responsibility to facilitate the best possible client recovery, it is also their responsibility to produce an outcome that reduces the need for future services and to accomplish this while utilizing the least amount of resources.

CLINICAL CASE MANAGEMENT TOOLS

To meet these responsibilities, therapists as individuals and the rehabilitation team as a whole have five clinical case management tools at their disposal:

1. Managing therapy resources:
   - Utilize only those disciplines that are absolutely necessary to achieve a client's expected outcome.
   - Provide only that frequency of each discipline's interventions that are absolutely necessary to achieve a client's expected outcome.
   - Provide the services of each discipline in the sequence that is absolutely necessary to achieve a client's expected outcome.
2. Managing treatment duration: ensure that each discipline provides its services only for the length of time that is absolutely necessary to achieve a client's expected outcome.
3. Managing the service delivery format: provide only that amount of individual therapy, group therapy, cotreatment, and therapy delivered by assistants and aides that is absolutely necessary to achieve a client's expected outcome.
4. Managing the level of care: ensure that services are only provided at the level of care (i.e., inpatient acute rehabilitation, skilled nursing

facility, home health, or outpatient) that is absolutely necessary to achieve a client's expected outcome.

5. Managing risks for complications: identify any physical, physiologic, psychologic, psychosocial, life style, and/or environmental factors that may impede a client's progress toward his or her expected outcome or cause regression from his or her achieved outcome after discharge, and take action during the course of rehabilitation to eliminate or reduce them.

MANAGING THERAPY RESOURCES

As discussed in Chapter 1, no external limits were placed on the type, frequency, and duration of services that could be provided in the fee-for-service era of rehabilitation. In 1976 the Health Care Financing Administration (HCFA) made an initial attempt to limit services when it instituted the so-called "three hour rule." The intention of this rule was to provide physicians and therapists with a tool to differentiate between those clients who required intensive multidisciplinary treatment and those who did not. In essence, this Medicare guideline indicated that admission to and continued stay in an acute rehabilitation program could only be justified if the client required an intensive multidisciplinary approach. Intensive was defined as a minimum of three hours of rehabilitation a day, which included physical therapy, occupational therapy, and/or speech therapy. Medicare's expectation was that providers would use this guideline to screen their prospective client admissions and admit only those who met it. The intention of this rule was not to suggest that all who needed rehabilitation should receive three hours of therapy a day. On the contrary, it was an attempt to reduce overutilization of therapy services. Providers did not respond in the expected manner, however. They adopted this rule as the service delivery model for rehabilitation. Within the context of this model, all clients requiring rehabilitation received a minimum of three hours of therapy per day. It was not long before private payers also adopted the requirement of three hours of therapy as their criterion for inpatient rehabilitation. The providers' action was the result of the absence of less intense levels of rehabilitation at that point in time. Over the ensuing years, therapists grew to accept this as the standard for resource utilization.

The managed care payment system requires therapists to move away from the almost reflexive expectation that all clients should receive three hours of therapy a day. Instead, therapists must engage in a clinical decision-making process that aligns the frequency, intensity, and duration of therapy with the prevailing needs and rehabilitation potential of the client at any given point in time during the course of rehabilitation.

To do this, the team uses three clinical decision-making tools to manage their resources:

1. Utilizing only those disciplines that are absolutely necessary to the attainment of expected outcomes
2. Sequencing discipline utilization across time in relation to the client's needs
3. Modulating the frequency and amount of disciplinary intervention

Utilizing Only Those Disciplines That Are Absolutely Necessary

The first step in managing resources is to determine which disciplines are required to ensure that the client attains his or her expected outcome. This clinical decision-making question applies not only to identifying the makeup of the team that will initiate treatment but also to determining which disciplines are absolutely required throughout the client's entire course of rehabilitation.

Even though a client may have a wide array of impairments, not all of them will prevent attainment of the projected outcome. Only those impairments that must be reduced in order to achieve the prevailing outcome should be treated and, consequently, only those disciplines that are required to treat these impairments should be utilized. The following are a few examples of this aspect of resource management.

Case Studies

RT is a retired firefighter who is post-left cerebrovascular accident (CVA) with residual right hemiplegia and moderate oral apraxia. After three weeks of treatment, the client had advanced in physical therapy from maximum to minimum assistant in transfers. At this point, the physical therapist determined that while the client could continue to improve his strength and balance, the degree of improvement would not be sufficient to move him to a lesser level of assistance. Thus, physical therapy was discontinued because the degree of improvement in strength and balance that would result from continued treatment would not change the client's level of disability.

*   *   *   *   *

MB is a 68-year-old homemaker who is post-left CVA with residual right hemiplegia and severe aphasia. After six weeks of treatment, the speech pathologist determined that she had successfully facilitated a functional communication system between the client and her spouse. The system consisted of a very limited repertoire of spoken words, which, combined with gestures and pointing to single printed words and/or pictures, allowed the client's husband to understand her needs and feelings. In the speech pathologist's opinion, the client had the potential to increase the number of single words she could say; however, this would not decrease the need for her and her husband to use the total communication system that they relied upon to communicate with ease. Further, in the speech pathologist's opinion, her own knowledge, skills, and judgment were not required to increase the number of words the client could speak. During the client's six weeks of treatment, her husband had been trained in techniques to facilitate the use of spoken words in the context of naturally occurring daily activities. The speech pathologist determined that the client could continue to improve with the assistance of her husband and discontinued treatment.

*   *   *   *   *

NR is a widowed householder who is post-right CVA with residual visual perceptual impairments, decreased left-sided sensation, and impulsiveness. The occupational therapist determined that the client's only impairments involved safety issues in the kitchen and when performing laundry and housecleaning tasks. The occupational therapist did not initiate treatment for this client, however, because she was to be discharged to a residential retirement facility that would provide for all of her meals, laundry, and housecleaning.

*   *   *   *   *

These cases illustrate an important clinical decision-making criterion relative to resource management: An impairment should be treated or continued to be treated only if the therapist has determined that treatment will either prevent secondary complications and/or significantly reduce the client's level of disability. The reduction of an impairment alone is insufficient clinical justification to initiate and/or continue treatment.

Sequencing Discipline Utilization

After identifying the necessary disciplines, the rehabilitation team's second resource management tool is to determine whether all team members should initiate treatment simultaneously or during different stages of the client's rehabilitation. The best point in time to initiate the services of the various disciplines varies among clients; there is no "one-size-fits-all" timing of rehabilitation interventions. The initiation of a given discipline's intervention should be based on three criteria: (1) prioritization of the client's needs, (2) a determination that the client has the physical and cognitive endurance necessary to participate in an intervention, and/or (3) whether or not the client has the cognitive ability to take advantage of a particular intervention.

Case Study

JK is a 32-year-old who was involved in a traffic accident in which a truck, traveling at 40 miles per hour, struck the rear of her stopped car. She is married, with a 2-year-old child, and is expecting a second child in six months. She was employed in a highly technical electronics job prior to the accident.

She has been diagnosed with a mild traumatic brain injury. Her impairments include the following:

- Moderate decrease of selective attention/concentration and short-term memory; inability to follow content of conversations, TV, or written material; or to remember where her child is, whether she has fed her child or herself, or whether she has turned off appliances ("It takes me 10 trips to the car to get everything in it that I need to take Melissa to the babysitter and go shopping.")
- Severely decreased endurance ("I must take a nap after every little thing I do . . . and I have to go to bed right after I fix dinner.")
- Severe intermittent headaches, cervical pain, dizziness, nausea ("I often spend most of the day in bed with the curtains closed.")

- Moderate decrease in frustration tolerance ("I get so easily upset and angry, I was never that way before, now just little things get me so upset, things that were so easy for me to do before.")
- Frequent mood swings

The client's greatest concern is the safety and care of her daughter and the proper care of herself for the health of her unborn child.

Client's treatment priority ranking. In discussing her problems with the case manager to determine the focus of her treatment, the client initially said that her attention and memory problems were her greatest concerns because she saw them posing the greatest threat to the safety and welfare of her children. As she and the case manager explored her daily routine, however, the client began to recognize a cascade effect between her headaches and pain, endurance, and her cognitive impairments. The headaches and pain caused her to stay in bed, which, in turn, further reduced her endurance. The headaches, pain, and low endurance together intensified her cognitive impairments, which led to a strong emotional reaction of inadequacy. This emotional stress consequently increased her headaches and pain. Realizing this interaction among her impairments, the client requested that the focus of her treatment program be prioritized in the following manner: (1) headaches and pain, (2) endurance, and (3) cognitive impairments.

In response to the client's request, the rehabilitation team decided that pain management through physical therapy and counseling should initially be the primary team focus. The team determined that speech therapy would only focus on compensatory cognitive strategies to address the safety issues and would be discontinued as soon as the client demonstrated the independent use of these strategies while her husband was at work. The team also decided that occupational therapy would not be utilized, since speech therapy would address the household management safety problems and the client did not present with other problems with activities of daily living (ADL). The team also decided that speech therapy would be resumed when the physical therapist and counselor determined that the client could manage her headaches and pain to such a degree that she would be able to benefit from treatment of her cognitive impairments. Stress management counseling would be decreased at this point to once a week for one month and then be scheduled on an as-needed basis. The team planned to phase in vocational counseling once the client's stress management counseling reached an as-needed level of intervention.

* * * * *

Modulating the Frequency and Amount of Disciplinary Intervention

The third resource management tool at the team's disposal is modulating or adjusting the frequency and amount of therapy that the client either requires or can tolerate. The number of times a client is treated per day or per week and the length of treatment time should be based on the priority of the client's needs and the client's endurance and/or cognitive ability to gain therapeutic advantage from intervention at any given point in time.

Case Study

JT is a 23-year-old college student majoring in electrical engineering who is post-traumatic brain injury with minimal left-sided weakness. He fluctuates cognitively between a confused and agitated state (Rancho Level 4) and a nonagitated confused state (Rancho Level 5). The client was primarily concerned about his inability to walk and engaged best in direct physical therapy treatment because of his vague awareness that this treatment was related to his inability to walk. Although he was not concerned with personal care and dressing problems, he did not resist occupational therapy because he recognized that this therapist was doing something for his weak arm and leg. He became the most confused and agitated with the speech-language pathologist because he could not tolerate direct demands on his cognitive abilities, nor could he see any reason to work with that therapist in less demanding ADL activities. Given these factors, the team decided that the client would receive physical therapy the greatest amount and length of the time, occupational therapy less frequently and for shorter periods of time, and therapeutic recreation intervention in the midafternoon and early evening when he could tolerate this level of cognitive challenge. The team decided against offering speech therapy at this time because the client's cognitive impairments could be addressed more effectively within the context of the other disciplines' treatment sessions.

* * * * *

MANAGING TREATMENT DURATION

The second clinical case management tool is managing the duration of treatment, the length of stay specified for each level of care. It is the therapist's responsibility to manage the rehabilitation process during that period in a manner that ensures attainment of the expected outcome during the specified length of stay. Management procedures include:

- establishing an expected outcome before treatment begins
- using critical pathways to monitor and problem solve client progress
- monitoring client progress on the basis of measurable and functional short-term goals that are directed toward attainment of the expected outcome

Establishing an Expected Outcome

The outcome is a statement that describes what the client will be able to do once impairments are reduced and/or certain skills have been regained. It is a description of the manner in which the client will be able to live. (See Exhibit 3–1.)

The outcome that the team selects is determined by three factors:

1. The client's clinical prognosis: Traditionally, therapists have projected a client's outcome solely on the basis of the type and severity of impairments and disabilities.

Exhibit 3–1 Example of Expected Outcomes

Outcome: Assisted Living
The client will be able to perform safely, completely, and accurately all usual and customary personal, household, community, and leisure activities of daily living with 25 percent or less daily physical, cognitive, and/or communicative assistance. The client will require a less demanding job.

Outcome: Modified Independent Living
The client will be able to perform all usual and customary personal, household, community, work, and leisure activities of daily living safely, completely, and accurately with that degree of assistance that normally occurs in the course of cooperative daily living. The client, however, will require a modified living and work environment, assistive devices/equipment, compensatory strategies, and/or more than the usual amount of time to complete tasks.

2. The client's health care benefits: Therapists must also consider the frequency, intensity, and duration of therapy that the client's health care plan will pay for. It is possible that the plan's benefits will not cover a level of treatment that will be required to reach an optimal outcome. In such cases, it is the therapist's responsibility to identify an outcome that can reasonably be achieved within the constraints of the therapy benefits allowed by the client's health insurance.

3. Providing rehabilitation at the least expensive level of care: Managed care payers and providers needing to keep client length of stay below PPS limits will want to move their clients to the least expensive level of care as quickly as possible. Thus, the rehabilitation team often finds itself establishing not the client's long-term outcome but rather the outcome required to transition the client's current level of care to the next less intense level of care. For example, a client admitted to inpatient acute rehabilitation may hold the ultimate prognosis of modified independent living. The team, however, selects assisted living. When that level is attained, the team transfers the client to a home and community-based level of care (a less expensive level of care than acute inpatient care) where rehabilitation will continue with the outcome goal now being modified independent living.

Working with Financial Constrains when Establishing Outcomes

To identify outcomes that can be achieved within different payer constraints, therapists must be well-acquainted with the different methods that various health plans and providers use to authorize treatment duration.

Indemnity Insurance. Indemnity insurance policies typically specify the number of physical therapy, speech therapy, occupational therapy, and psychology visits that are allowable per year. Notice the use of the word "allowable." The fact that a policy covers these services does not mean that the policyholder has free access to them. Prior approval from the insurance company must be obtained in order to access these benefits. When therapists are treating a client under an indemnity policy, they must be aware of how many visits have been approved and keep track of how many they have used. The insurer will not pay for any treatment beyond the authorized number of visits. If, at the end of the authorized treatment the client still has allowable visits remaining for that year, the provider's case manager can seek approval for additional visits. In the past, when the severity of a client's impairments, such as spinal cord injury or traumatic brain injury, required more treatment than allowed by the policy, the insurance company would "go out of plan." In this case, an insurance case manager would "substitute benefits" to obtain the funding for the amount of therapy needed. For example, if the client had skilled nursing facility care benefits, the amount of money allowed in the client's policy for those benefits would be used (substituted) for the needed rehabilitation services. While this occurs less frequently today, it remains an option. When it is available, the insurance company case manager will usually authorize an evaluation visit for each therapy discipline and request that a "proposed plan of care" be submitted at the end of the team evaluation. In addition to each discipline's findings, the proposed plan of care will also include the expected outcome of treatment and the projected frequency, intensity, and duration of treatment required by each discipline. The insurance case manager reviews the proposed plan of care and authorizes the level of services the insurance company deems necessary. The frequency and amount of therapy authorized may be that which was requested or less. Typically, therapy is authorized in 30-day periods of time at the end of which the case is reviewed and a determination made whether the client's progress warrants authorization of continued treatment.

Managed Care Plans. Most managed care plans "case manage" their clients. The managed care organization's (MCO) case manager or one that the MCO hires from a case management company specifies the number of inpatient days or outpatient visits authorized under preestablished MCO guidelines. MCOs do not "go out of plan." The case manager, however, in consultation with the MCO's primary care physician or utilization review committee can authorize additional days or visits if the clinical documentation indicates that continued treatment will result in further functional improvement.

Medicare. Medicare has different methods of authorizing treatment duration for inpatient and outpatient rehabilitation. A provider's TEFRA limit establishes the maximum duration of inpatient rehabilitation. Consequently, the provider (the therapist's employer) must inform the rehabilitation team of the maximum number of days allowed under that limit so they can select the outcome they believe can be achieved within that time frame. By the year 2000 or 2001, Medicare will use a PPS for inpatient rehabilitation.

For outpatient rehabilitation, a physician must certify the client's need for rehabilitation and recertify his or her ongoing need every 30 days. The certification and recertification substantiate the medical necessity for outpatient rehabilitation. The initial certification indicates that the client will make significant practical improvement in a reasonable and predictable period. The recertification signifies that the client has in fact made significant practical improvement during a specified 30-day period. This does not mean, however, that treatment is open-ended in the Medicare program. Outpatient rehabilitation services are subject to retrospective review by Medicare, which is based on the therapist's ongoing case documentation. If the documentation does not substantiate that the client made significant practical improvement during a given 30-day period, the Medicare reviewer will deny the claim and the provider will not be paid even though a physician has certified and recertified the need for rehabilitation. Consequently, the therapist must project the client's most probable outcome and terminate treatment immediately upon its attainment or upon determining that the client is not making significant practical improvement toward it. Beyond either of these points lies what Medicare refers to as "maintenance care," which is not a covered Medicare benefit.

Medicaid. Medicaid is a state and federal health care program that serves those under 65 years of age who cannot afford health care. In the Medicaid program, frequency and duration of treatment are determined by prior authorization. The provider submits a treatment authorization request (TAR), which indicates the diagnosis, treatment plan, and the number of visits requested by the therapist. The Medicaid reviewer authorizes the number of visits deemed necessary. Medicaid only authorizes for periods of 30 days. If the therapist believes continued treatment is warranted, another TAR must be submitted at least one week before the end of the previously authorized 30-day period to ensure continuity of care.

The outcome that the team selects should be one that they believe the client can achieve within the duration of treatment that has been approved by the payer. Thus, while a client may hold the prognosis of modified independent living, the outcome the team selects might be assisted living. When that level is attained, the team is then able to transfer the client to a home and community-based level of care where rehabilitation will continue with the outcome goal now being modified independent living. If the team determines at any time that the outcome will be a level of living that is lower than the client's current level of care, the team should immediately transfer the client to that level of care. For example, a client in a coma resulting from a traumatic brain injury is admitted to a subacute rehabilitation unit. The team initially decides that the client holds the potential to reach an outcome of admission to the acute inpatient rehabilitation level of care. After six weeks of rehabilitation, the client has not shown any signs of responding to this level of intervention. As a consequence, the team determines that the client's outcome is most likely that of total care and it recommends that the client be discharged to the long-term care unit of a skilled nursing facility. The expected outcome here would be that of physiologic maintenance (e.g., maintaining an adequate and safe system of nutrition, prevention of aspiration and contractures, and preservation of skin integrity). The skilled nursing facility staff would also monitor the client for a positive change in the client's neurologic status and request a reevaluation of rehabilitation potential if and when such a change in status occurs.

To obtain an extension of treatment duration, regardless of payer source, it is crucial that the therapist's documentation clearly and objectively demonstrates the type and degree of actual client improvement as well as the client's potential to make further significant gains as a result of continued therapy, at either the current or recommended level of care. Further, the type and degree of continued gains must also be objectively specified in the documentation. (See Chapter 8.)

Using Critical Pathways To Monitor and Problem Solve Client Progress

A map without a destination is as useless as a destination without a map. Absent a destination, one will randomly follow routes on a map with no knowledge of how long the journey will take nor of when the journey has been completed. With rehabilitation, the expected outcome is the destination and the critical pathway is the map that lays out the most appropriate and timely route leading to that destination. A *critical pathway* is a tool to monitor and problem solve client progress. It identifies the key rehabilitation activities that must occur and the times when they must occur in order to reach a preestablished outcome within a specified time period.

Critical pathways help the team achieve an expected outcome on a timely basis in two ways:

1. They speed up the rehabilitation process by reducing delays in service delivery. Typically, an organized treatment plan is not established and implemented until the first team conference. A critical pathway is, in effect, a team treatment plan that has been agreed upon even before the client arrives at the rehabilitation facility. As such, an outcome-directed organized team treatment plan can be implemented immediately upon a client's admission to the facility. The first team conference is then used to individualize the critical pathway. Because a critical pathway indicates what interventions should be occurring at specified times and what the expected client response to those interventions should be, therapists can immediately identify any variations from these expectations, problem solve them, and take corrective action. There is no need to wait for a scheduled conference to problem solve and establish an action plan. When a conference is held, the variations and action plans are discussed and revised if necessary.

2. Critical pathways increase the effectiveness of rehabilitation. They serve as a guidance mechanism to ensure that the team is providing the appropriate type of intervention at the proper time and that the intervention is producing the expected client outcomes. As such, they bring predictability and organization to interdisciplinary interventions and foster their coordination at the time of service delivery rather than at a conference that occurs sometime later. By setting forth clear, agreed-upon standards of rehabilitation, a critical pathway also reduces variations in treatment approaches and the sequence of treatment provisions that are related to differences in training or individual preferences. Finally, a critical pathway helps preserve continuity of care when staff changes occur during the course of a client's rehabilitation program. Because the sequence, timing, and response expectations are spelled out, a new therapist can easily step into the flow of treatment without spending hours poring through the medical record.

Development of a Critical Pathway

Critical pathways should be developed for the most common diagnoses treated in a given facility. At a minimum, a critical pathway should meet the following criteria:

- leads to a specific outcome
- identifies the key client performance domains that must be addressed
- identifies the typical phases of recovery that must occur for each client performance domain in order to reach the outcome
- identifies the length of each phase of recovery
- identifies the key interventions that must occur in each recovery phase
- identifies the expected changes in the client's abilities as a result of the key interventions during each recovery phase

The development process usually involves the steps outlined below:

- The provider establishes a task force of the disciplines that are most frequently involved in the direct provision of services to a particular diagnostic group.
- The task force establishes the most typical outcomes for the usual length of stay for that diagnostic group.
- The task force identifies the key client performance domains (e.g., ambulation, self-care, communication) that must be treated in order to achieve the outcomes.
- The task force conducts a chart review of discharged clients that reached the various outcomes to identify:
  1. the key interventions that occurred for each client performance domain and the average length of time from admission at which they occurred. Key interventions are those that are absolutely critical to progress; those that have proven either to affect progress adversely by their omission or positively by their commission.
  2. the typical change in the client's level of performance as a result of these key interventions
  3. the total length of time required to reach the outcome
- The task force prepares a rough draft of the critical pathway and solicits comments and suggestions from the larger group that provides direct services to the diagnostic group as well as from ancillary departments, such as pharmacy, lab, nutrition, orthotics, housekeeping, and unit clerks.
- The task force revises the critical pathway on the basis of the recommendations and returns it to the same broad group for review and, if necessary, continues to modify the critical pathway until there is a

consensus about the typical outcomes for the diagnostic group, the key interventions, and timing of therapy, as well as the changes in the client's level of performance that is expected in response to these interventions.

- The critical pathway is then used for a trial period and further refined on the basis of actual clinical experience.

A typical complete critical pathway covers the key areas of medical, nursing, therapy, and counseling interventions. Tables 3–1, 3–2, and 3–3 present examples of three subcomponents of a critical pathway—ambulation, self-care, and communication. As shown in these examples, the diagnostic group and expected outcome is specified at the top. The key client performance domains are indicated in the "Performance Area" column and the key interventions and the timing of them are listed in the following columns. The level of client performance that is expected to result from these interventions across time is shown at the bottom of these columns across from "Performance Level" in the "Performance Area" column. The expected outcome level of performance is indicated at the bottom of the "Expected Outcome" column. Critical pathways such as these lay out the treatment plan (key interventions) and short-term goals (expected performance levels) for the entire course of rehabilitation for the specified outcome before treatment even begins. With this tool, the team is able to manage treatment duration by knowing in advance what interventions must be provided, when they are to be provided and, most important, the level of client performance that should occur within the specified time frames. The critical factor in managing treatment duration is knowing the expected performance level, for if a client does not reach this level by the expected time, the team is immediately alerted to the presence of a problem that could prolong rehabilitation beyond its expected duration if not solved quickly. Finally, the example in the tables of a rehabilitation duration of 21 to 26 days does not necessarily mean that these critical pathways span one level of care. As soon as a client no longer requires immediate physician and nursing care, the client will be discharged either to a home health level of care or an outpatient level of care. This could occur as early as the second week of rehabilitation.

Table 3–1 Ambulation Component of Critical Pathway

Diagnosis: Left CVA; Outcome: Supervised Living

Performance Area	Admission	Week One (Day 1–6)	Week Two (Day 7–14)	Week Three (Day 15–20)	DC Day (Day 21–26)	Expected Outcome
Ambulation Intervention	• Assess motor control, fit and stand balance, tone, sensation, proprioception • Determine previous functional level • Determine current living environment • Determine pt. goals	• Assess upright status • Initiate treatment of identified problems including dissociation of head, trunk, and extremities; ability to assume standing; development of equal weight bearing and symmetry in standing; and development of weight shifting and balance in standing	• Assess • Develop selective voluntary control required for ambulation • Develop ability to use assistive device	• Ongoing • Evaluate and prescribe appropriate orthotic device PRN • Determine, write prescription, and order appropriate assistive device in consultation with patient/family ↕ Flight of 6 stairs	• Complete training • Complete assistive device training • Finalize adjustments to orthotic device PRN • Develop ability to don/doff device • Obtain appropriate equipment prior to discharge • Instruct family in guarding patient during ambulation PRN • Amb.- 100 ft.	
Expected Performance Level	Max. Assist	Mod. Assist	Min. Assist	Min. Assist	Supervised	Independent with single point care

Table 3–2 Self-Care Component of Critical Pathway

Diagnosis: Left CVA; Outcome: Supervised Living

Performance Area	Admission	Week One (Day 1–6)	Week Two (Day 7–14)	Week Three (Day 15–20)	DC Day (Day 21–26)	Expected Outcome
Self-Care Intervention	• Assess functional skills • Begin training patient in appropriate technique for self-care	• Ongoing • Ongoing • Introduce appropriate adaptive equipment for self-care and feeding	• Ongoing • Ongoing • Ongoing • Begin family/caregiver training of self-care techniques • Assess equipment needs and make recommendations	• Ongoing • Ongoing • Ongoing • Continue family/care training • Complete training prior to first LOA PRN • Ongoing	• Complete training • Reassess performance • Complete family/caregiver training • Finalize equipment needs • Issue/order appropriate equipment • Assess home management skills • Provide home management training as appropriate • Finalize discharge recommendation	
Performance Level						Mod. Indep/Supervised
Feeding	Min. Assist	Standby Assist	Set Up/Supervised	Set Up	Mod. Indep	
Hygiene Grooming	Min. Assist	Standby Assist	Set Up/Supervised	Set Up	Mod. Indep	
Bathing/Drsg:UEs	Mod. Assist	Min./Mod. Assist	Standby Assist	Set Up/Supervised	Supervised	
Bathing/Drsg:LEs	Max. Assist	Mod. Assist	Min. Assist	Standby Assist	Supervised	
Toileting	Max. Assist	Mod. Assist	Min. Assist	Standby Assist	Supervised	

Table 3–3 Communication Component of Critical Pathway

Diagnosis: Left CVA; Outcome: Supervised Living

Performance Area	Admission	Week One (Day 1–6)	Week Two (Day 7–14)	Week Three (Day 15–20)	DC Day (Day 21–26)	Expected Outcome
Communication Intervention	• Assess communication • Initiate communication system for basic needs PRN • Adjust environment to include appropriate call system PRN	• Ongoing • Implement treatment program and family/caregiver education • Provide recommendations to staff • Begin family/caregiver training	• Ongoing • Continue with treatment program and family/caregiver education	• Ongoing • Reevaluation	• Ongoing • Complete treatment program and family/caregiver training	
Expected Performance Level	Receptive Mod. Assist Expressive-Max. Assist	Receptive Min. Assist Expressive-Max. Assist	Receptive Standby Assist Expressive-Mod. Assist	Receptive Modified Ind. Expressive-Min./Mod. Assist	Receptive Mod. Assist Expressive-Min. Assist	Receptive Modified Ind. Expressive-Min. Assist

MANAGING SERVICE DELIVERY FORMAT

The third clinical case management tool used by the rehab team to manage the quality and cost of rehabilitation is managing how services are provided. Historically, therapy has been provided primarily in a one-on-one (individual therapy) service delivery format. This was regarded as the most effective manner of treating a client's problems and, therefore, was equated with the highest quality of care. Alternative service delivery formats such as group therapy, cotreatment, and use of aides were often viewed as providing a lesser quality of care. Nontraditional means of providing treatment, such as the use of family members, caregivers, peers, and community volunteers were rarely, if ever, deemed appropriate. These assumptions were reinforced by the fee-for-service payment structure, which is based on an individual therapy service delivery model. There was a time in which group therapy was not a reimbursable service delivery format, and even today it is not recognized in many indemnity insurance payment systems. Payers have viewed cotreatment as a duplication of services and they will not pay for family education and training. Because of these payment biases, therapists were not challenged in the past to identify additional methods of providing therapy, methods that could produce results equal to individual therapy. The therapist's bias toward a one-on-one service delivery format is being challenged in the managed care environment. Because individual therapy is the most expensive service delivery format, managed care is challenging therapists to identify equally effective alternatives and employ them when clinically appropriate. At certain points in time and for varying durations, all patients require individual therapy. All patients, however, do not require individual therapy all the time in order to attain their expected outcome. Cotreatment, group therapy, supervised independent therapy, and the use of aides, family/caregivers, peers, or volunteers represent a broad menu of potential service delivery formats in addition to individual therapy. The determination of the best service delivery format for a given client must be based on whether the client meets preestablished admission criteria for each of these modes of service delivery that are established by each discipline. (See Exhibit 3–2.)

Using these admission criteria, the therapist and/or team selects the service delivery format they believe will produce the best results for the least cost during the course of rehabilitation. A client's service delivery format should never be selected solely on the basis of reducing cost and/or

Exhibit 3–2 Example of Group Therapy and Cotreatment Admission Criteria

1. The client's evaluation has been completed and the outcome, short-term goals, and treatment plan have been established.
2. The client exhibits an emerging awareness and control of his or her emotional status.
3. Group therapy is used when:
   a. Two or more clients have similar diagnoses, goals, treatment activities, levels of physical independence, levels of cognitive independence, and functional experience needs.
   b. Two or more clients have dissimilar diagnoses but complementary strengths and weaknesses.
   c. Two or more clients have dissimilar diagnoses but complementary needs and abilities.
4. Cotreatment is used when:
   a. The client cannot tolerate two separate hours of treatment from each discipline but can tolerate two disciplines during the same hour.
   b. The client requires a treatment approach that will help him or her to understand and apply the interrelating skills that each discipline is working on separately.
   c. The therapists need a practical hands-on medium to learn how to carry over and reinforce each other's goals in their respective individual and/or group therapy sessions.

increasing productivity; on the contrary, it should be one that the therapist has determined will facilitate the greatest improvement, in the least amount of time, for the least cost.

Group Therapy

Group therapy can be a very powerful treatment approach. It holds the potential to increase a client's rate of learning and self-monitoring skills. Not only does each group member receive some individual intervention during a group treatment, but he or she can also observe the therapist and/ or an aide working with other members. The ability to observe the actions and hear the dialogue between the therapist and other group members indirectly provides continuous reinforcement of approaches to task performance. By observing and listening, the clients are provided with the opportunity to think through and practice a task performance independently. Peer interaction and feedback encourages self-monitoring. Group therapy also has a number of other benefits: It provides an opportunity for feedback from the therapist and group members in a climate of acceptance and support. Such a climate encourages self-initiation of therapy procedures and decreases the client's perception that the therapist will "cure me" which, in turn, decreases the client's dependence on the therapist. Finally, group therapy provides a forum in which to teach carryover and generalization of that which has been taught in individual therapy.

Group therapy, based on sound clinical admission and discharge criteria, as well as appropriate treatment procedures, can be a powerful quality and cost management tool. It can result in the more rapid application of a new skill outside of the therapy environment which, in turn, may lead to the use of that skill in the context of related tasks that have not been directly addressed in therapy (e.g., generalization of skills). Independent skill generalization can lead to a more durable outcome. The faster a client learns and generalizes a skill the shorter will be the length of stay in treatment. Costs are controlled by achieving the expected outcome in the shortest possible time and producing an outcome that is durable. These quality and cost-control benefits will not be realized, however, if management mandates group treatment as a means of reducing costs by treating more clients per day with fewer staff. The absence of appropriate clinical decision making will nullify any perceived costs savings. The rate of client progress will not be increased and the outcome will not be as durable.

Levels of Group Therapy

For group therapy to be effective, a client must be placed in a group that is designed to meet his or her specific types of needs. Group therapy usually encompasses one of these three areas: impairment reduction, skill reinforcement, and skill generalization.

Impairment reduction group. All patients in this group have similar therapeutic needs, receive the same type of therapy, and require the direct, hands-on facilitation and guidance of a therapist and/or aide. All patients do not have to be at the same level of impairment, however (e.g., oral motor exercise group, visual neglect/visual field cut group, active upper extremity range of motion group).

Admission criteria for such a group would be clients who require moderate physical, cognitive, and/or communicative assistance to participate in and complete treatment activities safely and accurately.

Skill reinforcement group. Clients in this group have reached the level of skill accuracy and consistency in individual therapy where they no longer require the constant direct intervention and guidance of a therapist to ensure safe and accurate responses. These clients are at the point where they require repetitive practice of a skill (e.g., safe transfer techniques, visual scanning of right visual fields, word retrieval strategies) to ensure its permanency. Clients in this group require task setup, monitoring for accuracy, and intervention if unsafe and/or inaccurate responses begin to emerge. The role of the group therapist is to assist and guide the client through the performance of skills within the context of functional tasks. In a skill reinforcement group, the therapy exists more in the clients' actual performance of tasks than from hands-on intervention of a therapist.

Admission criteria for this type of group includes clients who require task setup and standby physical, cognitive, and/or communicative assistance to participate in and complete treatment activities safely and accurately.

Skill generalization. In this group, the clients practice newly gained skills within the context of real-life functional activities (cooking, communicating with community businesses by telephone, safe mobility on all surfaces and in crowds). Members of the group work toward individual and/or group goals within the context of a functional activity. During the activity, the clients monitor their own performance as well as provide feedback to each other regarding the effectiveness of their approach to the activity. The role of the therapist is to coach, monitor, and offer feedback to reinforce what the client is doing well and encourage individual and group evaluation of why something is not being done well and how it might be changed.

Admission criteria include clients who require activity setup and periodic monitoring and feedback to participate and complete the treatment activity safely and accurately.

Group Size and Degree of Homogeneity

The number of clients in a group and the diversity of types of impairments and skills being treated can be increased as one moves through the impairment reduction, skill reinforcement, and skill generalization phases of treatment. Typically there are no more than four clients in an impairment reduction group unless it is staffed by two personnel, in which case five to six clients could be treated effectively. At the skill reinforcement level, four to five clients can be treated effectively by one person and six by two staff. When the skill generalization level is reached, six clients could be treated effectively by one person and seven to eight by two staff.

Staffing Patterns

The impairment reduction level is typically staffed by a single discipline while the next two levels lend themselves to a cotreatment service delivery format. When two staff are required at any of the three levels of treatment, then one person should be an aide unless it is a cotreatment format.

Cotreatment

The traditional individual therapy format of treatment tends to be fragmented. The client sees the physical therapist for one aspect of a problem, the speech-language pathologist for another, and occupational therapist for still another. Each discipline has its own goals and often it is left to the client to determine how the various goals and treatments work together to achieve the expected outcome. A cotreatment service delivery format provides the therapists with the opportunity to demonstrate to the client how their separate goals interrelate and how the different treatments interlock to support movement toward a common outcome goal. Co-treatment also affords the therapists the opportunity to observe the client in a different functional context, which often reveals both positive and negative performance characteristics that may be hidden when focusing the client on only one aspect of a problem. This information can help the therapist to refine the treatment approaches of each discipline further to meet the client's needs and capabilities. This method of service delivery also allows the therapists to gain a better understanding of each others' goals and treatment approaches.

Cotreatment does not directly reduce cost since the cost of two therapists is the same whether services are provided sequentially or conjointly. It does have a positive indirect cost reduction affect, however, in that a client's length of treatment will be shortened through a more rapid understanding of the purpose of treatment and an enhanced ability to meet performance expectations.

Cross Training

Two or more disciplines treating a client at the same time offer three powerful treatment advantages. Cotreatment can act to decrease the fragmentation of service, provide therapists an opportunity to observe and learn about their client in a variety of functional demand settings, and facilitate discipline cross training.

Client needs rarely fit the historic segmented rehabilitation service delivery format in which the client receives individual treatment for physical therapy, occupational therapy, speech-language therapy, or counseling in separate locations within the rehabilitation facility. While therapists segment the client's impairments, the client does not. Clients bring all of their impairments to all locations in the facility—they bring the totality of all their needs to every caregiver in the facility. For this reason, all therapists and nursing personnel should be capable of responding to and assisting clients with all their needs at some level of skill. "Cross training" places each therapist in a position to reinforce each others' treatment approaches when they work with a client in their respective individual treatment sessions. For example, in one stroke rehabilitation program, all team members are cross trained in transfers, positioning, active range of motion, dysphagia feeding techniques, stress management, and methods to facilitate and reinforce communication. Each team member is responsible for responding to client needs in these areas as they arise. For example, if a wheelchair-dependent client needs to use the bathroom during a speech therapy session, the speech-language pathologist does not make the client wait, stop the treatment session, or call a nurse. Instead, the speech-language pathologist takes the client to the bathroom and facilitates the transfer. If and when appropriate, the speech-language pathologist also uses this as an opportunity to continue treatment in the context of a functional activity. In another instance, a physical therapist, who has dysphagia training, could work on sitting balance and posture at meal times while simultaneously facilitating and monitoring safe swallowing techniques. In this manner the "cross-trained" speech-language pathologist and physical therapist bring their treatment into the client's natural environment and treat in the context of a real-life need and activity. This increases the client's rate of learning and the durability of the outcome because the skill has been acquired in the context of a natural activity. In this context, cross training holds the potential to increase quality of care through increased frequency and continuity of treatment, which, in turn, can potentially decrease a client's length of stay and increase the durability of an outcome. Both decreased length of stay and outcome durability decrease the cost of rehabilitation.

Use of Rehabilitation Aides

As therapists assume the clinical case manager's role and pressure mounts to find less expensive means of providing services, rehabilitation aides will be used increasingly to supplement therapist-provided treatment. Regardless of their discipline, therapists will be asked to identify components of a client's condition that do not require the skills of a therapist for safe, appropriate, and effective treatment. Similarly, therapists will be asked to identify stages in the recovery process where an aide can as effectively facilitate patient progress as a therapist.

In the coming years, therapists will triage their clients into the following four categories:

1. clients who only require a therapist to evaluate their condition, establish the goals and treatment plan, and monitor an aide's provision of the plan to ensure appropriate and effective treatment
2. clients who require a therapist to evaluate their case, establish the treatment plan, provide the initial phase of treatment, and evaluate the client's response to the treatment plan and modify it to ensure its appropriateness and effectiveness. Once the therapist is satisfied with the treatment plan and the client's response to it, the client is transitioned to an aide who carries out the plan under the therapist's supervision.
3. clients who require the ongoing treatment of a therapist for certain complex aspects of care and the ongoing intervention of an aide for other less complex aspects of care
4. clients who have such a highly complex case that the therapist is the primary service provider throughout the major course of rehabilitation, with the aide providing supplementary therapy

Regardless which group a client is assigned, the therapist will intervene at preestablished stages to reassess the client's progress toward treatment goals and modify the treatment plan as indicated. The therapist remains responsible for continually monitoring the client's progress and determining when it would be appropriate to transition clients who initially were in groups 3 and 4 into group 1 level of care.

The utilization of aides should be based upon clinical criteria, established by therapists, that identify when, how, and with whom aide intervention will be safe and effective. At a minimum, such criteria could be based on the distinction between skilled therapist services and nonskilled aide services.

Skilled vs. Nonskilled Services

Payers define skilled services as those requiring the knowledge, skills, and judgment of a therapist for the treatment and amelioration of impairments and disabilities caused by a medical condition.

- Knowledge is a course of academic preparation specifically related to the services required by the medical condition.
- Skills are a specific array of technical assessment and treatment interventions appropriate to each population served that are acquired through an academic and clinical training program followed by a supervised clinical affiliation and continuing education and clinical experience.
- Judgment is the ability to apply professional practice standards when deciding whether a given client requires intervention, and, if so, which knowledge and skills are required to treat a given condition appropriately and when treatment should be discontinued.

Within this context, nonskilled aide patient care services are those that can be safely and effectively rendered without a specialized academic degree and skills acquired through an academic and clinical training program. To develop and implement the aide level of care, each discipline must complete the following steps for each diagnostic group:

1. Identify client conditions. Each therapy discipline must establish clinical criteria that identify and distinguish between patient conditions that absolutely require the knowledge, skills, and judgment of a therapist to ensure patient safety as well as progress toward an attainment of the expected outcome versus those patient conditions

that can be treated by an aide with equal assurance of patient safety and progress.

2. Identify timing of aide intervention. Each discipline must establish clinical criteria by diagnosis and/or specific impairments that identify the appropriate time at which services should be transitioned from therapist to aide or aide to therapist.
3. Identify tasks and procedures. Each discipline needs to identify specific tasks, techniques, and routines that can be provided by an aide and configure them into standardized aide treatment protocols for each diagnosis and/or impairment. The treatment protocols should also include criteria for the discontinuation of a treatment procedure and the request for therapist assistance to ensure the safety and welfare of the patient.

Nontraditional Service Providers: Family/Caregivers, Peers, and Community Volunteers

Family/Caregiver Service Providers

Historically, families and caregivers have received education and training regarding the purpose, goals, and supervision of home programs. With ever decreasing lengths of stay, however, it is often necessary to provide the family/caregiver with specific treatment techniques that are necessary to facilitate continued improvement after discharge. Many clients reach the point in therapy at which they hold the potential for continued improvement but no longer require the knowledge, skills, and judgment of a therapist to achieve their objectives. Such clients, however, do require someone who can consistently and repetitively facilitate and encourage the client's performance of treatment tasks, techniques, and routines to realize their potential. Other clients reach a point in therapy at which, in the therapist's opinion, they do not hold the potential for further improvement. Yet these clients also require someone to facilitate their continued performance of techniques and routines in order to maintain the level of function they have attained.

Family members should be trained to carry out treatment techniques that will either facilitate continued improvement or maintain existing skills. They should be screened prior to training however, to ensure that they possess the emotional, physical, and cognitive strength and endurance required for this role. For working family members, therapists should also determine whether they can realistically provide the amount and/or timing of the required intervention in the time they have available before or after work. Nonfamily caregivers should be trained and utilized when the family member does not meet any of these pretraining criteria.

To be successful, family education and training must address two frequent and significant barriers to a family member's willingness to assume the role of a service provider. First, some hold the perception that it is the therapist's responsibility to treat and "cure" the client. Their perception is that, "I am paying you to provide the service and should not have to be responsible for any aspect of treatment or care." The second barrier arises when a family believes the client will recover completely. In such instances, the family feels little need to put forth effort in facilitating skills that won't be needed later. In this instance, all attempts to educate and train family members prior to discharge are resisted and often yield further requests for continued or more intense therapy. Neither of these barriers can be overcome in the last weeks of treatment. (See Chapter 6.) Education, counseling, and training must begin from the moment of admission to the rehabilitation program and occur in small doses through-out the course of the client's rehabilitation. Further, most of this family intervention must occur in the context of the client's treatment sessions rather than at a family conference. When education and training is pro-vided during a treatment session, the family member can raise questions and concerns at the moment they are attempting to learn a particular technique. Since the client and the family member are learning during the course of rehabilitation, the family member should be encouraged to attend as many therapy sessions as possible. This gives both the therapist and family member the opportunity to discuss attitudes, perceptions, and beliefs on an ongoing basis. This continual dialogue, rather than a single conference, has a greater probability of lowering the barriers to a family's acceptance of its role in rehabilitation.

Volunteer Peer Coaching

Individuals with personal experience of a catastrophic illness or injury and subsequent rehabilitation can often provide valuable assistance to others who are undergoing rehabilitation treatment. Such individuals, for example, could provide real-life coaching tips related to topics such as:

- use and updating of memory books
- safety awareness
- compensating for visual perceptual impairments
- energy conservation
- the importance of correct body mechanics
- stress management
- pain management
- adjustment to discharge from rehabilitation
- adjustment to disability

Community Volunteers and Community-Based Activity Programs

Certain clients may be at risk for decline in function because of the lack of companionship and lack of access to leisure activities. Volunteers drawn from sources such as friends, places of worship, or service clubs could be used to fill this need. Many communities offer a variety of productive activity programs at minimal or no cost. Libraries, religious organizations, and museums frequently hold lecture series or discussion groups. Senior and youth centers offer a wide variety of activities, as do the parks and recreations departments of most cities. Adult classes at local high schools and community colleges provide opportunities to pursue certain hobbies, participate in craft classes, or engage in intellectual activities. While these activity programs are not specifically designed for people with disabilities, they can provide a rich environment that can stimulate and maintain a client's abilities after discharge from rehabilitation. Prior to discharge from rehabilitation, clients should receive information regarding the value, location, and means of accessing the productive activity programs that are available in their community. The use of community volunteers and community-based activity programs should be part of the client's discharge plan. The appropriate member or members of the therapy team are responsible for identifying and training the volunteers or for linking the client and the client's family with the community-based activity program prior to discharge.

MANAGING THE LEVEL OF CARE

The fourth clinical management tool is ensuring that rehabilitation is being provided at the right level of care. Levels of care refer to the place in which rehabilitation services are rendered. The most common are inpatient acute medical units, acute inpatient rehabilitation hospitals or units within an acute care hospital, subacute units, skilled nursing facilities, home-based rehabilitation programs, and day rehabilitation programs.

Determining the Appropriate Level of Care

The initial determination of the appropriate level of care is typically made by the MCO's or insurance company's case manager in consultation with the client's primary care physician (PCP). This decision is based on the PCP's evaluation of the client's current medical status, type and degree of impairments that require rehabilitation, and the client's rehabilitation potential. The PCP uses these criteria to place the client at a level of care that is the least expensive and most medically appropriate. It would be unusual, however, for a client's rehabilitation to be completed at this initial level of care. The payer's expectation is that the client will be moved to successively less expensive levels of care as rapidly as possible. Thus, while the therapist or team typically does not play a role in determining the initial level of care, they do have a pivotal role in level of care decisions thereafter. The therapist or team will be responsible for identifying the point at which a client can be transferred to a less intense (i.e., costly) level of care without adversely affecting progress.

Case Study

For example, Joe, a 21-year-old college engineering student was admitted in a comatose state to the subacute unit of a rehabilitation hospital following a traumatic brain injury suffered in an automobile accident. After three weeks, he reached the confused and agitated phase of cognitive recovery and was moved to the acute rehabilitation unit. Although he could now tolerate a more intense rehabilitation program, he still required more intensive supervision for his safety. Joe had a minimal right hemiparesis and was at risk for a fall due to his attempts to walk while still in a confused state. Two weeks later, he was no longer agitated and his confusion had diminished to the point where he could safely continue his rehabilitation program at home with daytime supervision from a paid caregiver and with nighttime supervision provided by his parents. The caregiver also carried out rehabilitation techniques, provided by the therapists, in the context of Joe's performance of his daily living activities. Four weeks later, Joe had reached the point at which he could cognitively participate in and gain therapeutic advantage from an intensive outpatient rehabilitation program. At this time, he entered the hospital's day treatment program. After two months in this program, he was ready for a local community college program specially designed for individuals with traumatic brain injury, but based on an education model that was more in keeping with his goal of returning to school.

* * * * *

To participate in the decision-making process, therapists must know not only the admission and discharge criteria for the level of care at which they practice, but also the admission criteria for all other levels of care. With this knowledge, the therapist can evaluate a client's level of function at any given point in time in relationship to the admission criteria of a less intense level of care and determine when the client is ready for the next level of rehabilitation.

The various levels of care are not laid out in a continuum through which all rehabilitation clients pass. Clients will not necessarily move from the acute care medical unit to inpatient acute rehabilitation and then to a home-based treatment setting with outpatient rehabilitation as their final destination. Instead of a continuum, one may view the various levels of care as a menu (Figure 3–1) from which the most appropriate level of rehabilitation is selected at a given point in time based on client needs and abilities. This decision-making process begins at the level of the inpatient acute medical unit. Depending upon a client's level of medical care needs and the severity of his or her impairments, the client may be discharged from the acute medical unit either to inpatient acute or subacute rehabilitation, a skilled nursing facility (SNF), a home health agency, outpatient rehabilitation (either interdisciplinary team program or a single-discipline service), or to a long-term care facility if the client has no potential to benefit from rehabilitation. After discharge from the acute medical unit, the next

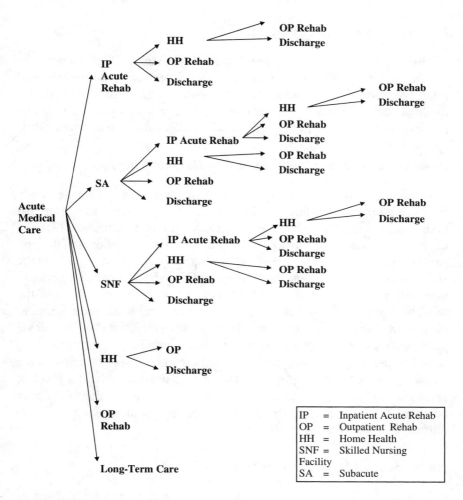

Figure 3–1 Levels of Care Menu

---

rehabilitation unit must make the next level of care decision. They must decide whether the client has reached his or her maximum potential and should be discharged from rehabilitation or whether the client holds the potential for further improvement and should be discharged to the next most appropriate level of care.

The following are general admission criteria to the various levels of care that the team can use to make these decisions.[2]

Inpatient Acute Medical Care Unit

This level of care includes rehabilitation services that are rendered in general acute care hospitals, medical/surgical units, trauma centers, and intensive care units. In these settings, the focus is on stabilizing the client's medical status and taking preventive measures such as passive range of motion, positioning, splinting, and swallowing evaluation and treatment.

Acute Inpatient Rehabilitation Hospital/Hospital Unit

Appropriate clients for this level of care are those who: (1) are medically fragile, requiring the immediate availability of a physician as well as 24-hour nursing support, (2) have severe functional impairments, and (3) have the potential to benefit from a coordinated intensive (three hours of therapy per day, six days per week) team rehabilitation program in order to make significant and timely gains from rehabilitation. The purpose of rehabilitation at this level of care is the prevention of complications and the reduction and/or compensation for impairments and functional limitations. The focus of rehabilitation here is only on facilitating that level performance of personal activities of daily living (e.g., toileting, transfers, mobility, dressing, and feeding) that is required to transfer the client home as safely and quickly as possible. Depending upon the client's level of ability at the time of transfer and his or her prognosis, the client may continue rehabilitation either through a home health agency or in an outpatient rehabilitation program.

Hospital-Based Subacute Rehabilitation

This level of care is appropriate for two types of clients, both of whom require 24-hour nursing care and immediate physician availability:

1. Those who do not require the intensity of an inpatient acute rehabilitation program in order to be discharged either to the next appropriate level of care or from rehabilitation altogether. The rehabilitation focus for this type of client is on the prevention of complications, the reduction of impairments, and the facilitation of functional skills.
2. Those whose medical status and/or endurance will not allow them to maximally benefit from intensive inpatient rehabilitation but are thought to hold that potential. The focus of rehabilitation for this type

of client is on prevention of complications until he or she is medically and/or physically able to participate in a more intensive level of rehabilitation. Intensive therapy, however, does not necessarily mean admission to inpatient acute rehabilitation. It may be determined that the client can achieve an optimal outcome in a home-based rehabilitation program or in an outpatient day rehabilitation program or other outpatient levels of care.

Skilled Nursing Facility

This level of care is appropriate for three different types of clients:

1. those who require 24-hour nursing care, do not require immediate physician availability, and can benefit from an intensive (three hours per day, six days a week) rehabilitation program. The rehabilitation focus for these clients is the same as inpatient acute rehabilitation. The only difference is that this type of client is not medically unstable and, therefore, does not require the immediate availability of a physician.
2. those who require 24-hour nursing care, do not require immediate physician availability, have the potential for significant functional improvement, but who cannot tolerate intensive rehabilitation and whose rate of improvement is expected to be in monthly rather than biweekly time increments. The focus of rehabilitation here is on prevention of complications and therapy to reduce impairments and functional limitations provided at a frequency and intensity within the client's level of endurance. (See Chapter 4 for definition of impairments, functional limitations, and disabilities.)
3. those who require 24-hour nursing care, do not require immediate physician availability, and whose rate of recovery is expected to be either greater than monthly or highly questionable. The focus of rehabilitation is intermittent single-discipline intervention. The purpose of the intervention is to establish a maintenance program designed to prevent complications as well as to support the client's existing level of function. The therapist trains nursing personnel and family members in the implementation of the maintenance program and periodically reevaluates the client to assess rehabilitation potential and modify the maintenance program as indicated.

Home- and Community-Based Rehabilitation

Home-based rehabilitation is typically provided through a home health agency. Clients appropriate for this level of care are those who are medically stable and only require as-needed physician care, but who do require an initial period of nursing care or supervision and intermittent care thereafter. These clients hold the potential for significant functional gains but do not require daily rehabilitation to realize them. They, do, however, need a coordinated team approach.

The focus of rehabilitation at this level of care continues to be on the reduction of and/or compensation for impairments and functional limitations in order to increase the client's level of independence in performing personal activities of daily living and to facilitate transfer to outpatient rehabilitation. This level of care, however, also begins to address the disability level, since the client's treatment is more frequently carried out in the context of functional daily living tasks. Home-based rehabilitation for non-Medicare clients may not be limited by the "homebound" rule. When this is the case, rehabilitation efforts can focus more extensively on the reduction of disabilities through the facilitation of functional skills within the context of the patient's real-life home and community needs and activities. Home-based rehabilitation for Medicare clients is allowable as long as the client is "homebound."[3] Homebound status is defined as follows: "a beneficiary will be considered to be homebound if he has a condition due to an illness or injury which restricts his ability to leave his place of residence except with the aid of supportive devices such as crutches, canes, wheelchairs, and walkers, the use of special transportation, or the assistance of another person or if he has a condition which is such that leaving his home is medically contraindicated."[4] This section also allows some treatment to occur in the community. It states that: "If the patient does in fact leave the home, the patient may nevertheless be considered homebound if the absences from the home are infrequent or for periods of relatively short duration, or are attributable to the need to receive medical treatment."[5]

Day Rehabilitation Program

This level of care is appropriate for those who hold the potential for significant functional improvement and require as-needed nursing and/or physician care. Clients at this level of care are those who can benefit from intensive (three to five days a week for three to six hours a day) interdisciplinary rehabilitation. The focus of rehabilitation at this level is the facilitation of functional skills that are specific to the needs and demands of the patient's living environment. These services may be provided in a hospital outpatient department, a comprehensive outpatient rehabilitation facility, or a free-standing outpatient rehabilitation facility.

MANAGING THE RISKS FOR COMPLICATIONS

Managing the risk for complications is the fifth clinical case management tool used by the rehabilitation team to manage the quality and cost of rehabilitation. Prevention of complications during the course of rehabilitation has long been understood as a critical factor in ensuring the best possible outcome in the shortest length of time. Therapists recognize that measures taken to prevent skin breakdown, protect joint integrity, and provide proper nutrition and hydration are as important to a client's timely and successful outcome as the therapeutic interventions provided. It is equally important for the team to take steps to prevent complications after discharge from rehabilitation. Outcome studies have identified problems such as preventable secondary medical complications, adjustment problems upon returning to home and community, and self-imposed social isolation.[6] Additionally, decline or absence of the use of one's home exercise programs that were provided by each discipline, improper medication management, improper exercise, and nutrition are also postdischarge complications. Clearly, complications such as these can, in short order, completely undo the gains made by a client during rehabilitation. Regression from the discharge level of functioning is costly from both a quality of life and fiscal perspective. As complications arise, the client's and family's hopes are dashed as previously attained skills erode and the family's level of caregiver burden increases. This situation usually intensifies rapidly because it occurs outside of the support and guidance of the rehabilitation team. From a fiscal standpoint, postdischarge complications can compound financial costs. Not only will the money expended to achieve the original outcome be lost but costs beyond this original expenditure will be substantially increased when the client must reenter the health care system in some manner.

The rehabilitation team holds a responsibility to identify those clients who are at risk for postdischarge complications and to include a plan of action in the client's treatment plan that will address them during the course of rehabilitation. Postdischarge follow-up of clients who are at risk for complications also is usually required to avert regression from the outcome achieved from rehabilitation.

CONCLUSION

The expanded roles and responsibilities of therapists individually, and the team as a whole, require them to produce the most effective (highest quality) rehabilitation outcome for a given client in the most efficient (least costly) manner. This chapter has presented the concept that quality and cost management are not mutually exclusive endeavors. When done correctly, cost management does not lead to decreased quality of care. Clinical decisions drive cost. Effective cost management, then, arises from sound clinical judgment and appropriate resource utilization decisions. In essence, the therapist and team can effectively manage quality and cost of service by appropriately managing their clinical resources, the duration of each disciplines' interventions, their service delivery format, the level of care in which the services are provided, and risk for complications. These five areas of clinical case management represent *what* must be managed during rehabilitation. The next step is to define *how* to manage them. A formalized clinical decision-making system that is utilized by all team members is a prerequisite to successful clinical case management. The Managed Outcome Rehabilitation (MOR) system, which will be presented in the next four chapters, provides such a formalized system.

REFERENCES

1. A. Schwab, Repositioning for Managed Care, *Rehab Management* Feb/March (1994): 81–83.
2. T. Goldsmith, *Managing Managed Care: A Practical Guide for Audiologists and Speech-Language Pathologists* (Rockville, MD: American Speech-Language-Hearing Association, 1994).
3. Health Care Financing Administration, *Home Health Agency Manual*, Pub. 11, Rev. 277 (Washington, DC: GPO, 1996), Section 204.1.
4. Health Care Financing Administration, *Home Health Agency Manual*.
5. Health Care Financing Administration, *Home Health Agency Manual*.
6. S. Forer, How To Make Program Evaluation Work for You, *Neurorehabilitation 2*, no. 4 (1992): 81–83.

CHAPTER 4

Client Management Tools

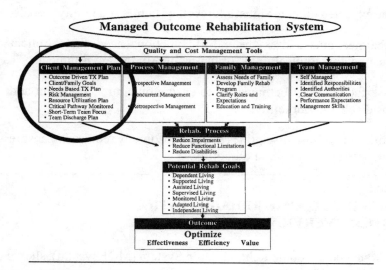

Managed Outcome Rehabilitation System

Quality and Cost Management Tools

Client Management Plan	Process Management	Family Management	Team Management
• Outcome Driven TX Plan • Client/Family Goals • Needs Based TX Plan • Risk Management • Resource Utilization Plan • Critical Pathway Monitored • Short-Term Team Focus • Team Discharge Plan	• Prospective Management • Concurrent Management • Retrospective Management	• Assess Needs of Family • Develop Family Rehab Program • Clarify Roles and Expectations • Education and Training	• Self Managed • Identified Responsibilities • Identified Authorities • Clear Communication • Performance Expectations • Management Skills

Rehab. Process
• Reduce Impairments
• Reduce Functional Limitations
• Reduce Disabilities

Potential Rehab Goals
• Dependent Living
• Supported Living
• Assisted Living
• Supervised Living
• Monitored Living
• Adapted Living
• Independent Living

Outcome
Optimize
Effectiveness   Efficiency   Value

Client Management Plan

- Outcome Driven TX Plan
- Client/Family Goals
- Needs Based TX Plan
- Risk Management
- Resource Utilization Plan
- Critical Pathway Monitored
- Short-Term Team Focus
- Team Discharge Plan

KEY POINTS

- The purpose of rehabilitation is to reduce functional limitations and disabilities.

- An expected outcome must be established before rehabilitation commences.

- The expected outcome must address the client's and family's goals.

- Treatment must address the real-life functional needs that the client must be able to meet in his or her natural living environment.

- Risk factors must be managed to ensure outcome attainment and postdischarge durability.

- Utilize only those disciplines that are absolutely required to ensure outcome attainment and durability.

MANAGED OUTCOME REHABILITATION SYSTEM OVERVIEW

The Managed Outcome Rehabilitation System (MORsystem), shown in Figure 4–1, provides the team with a set of quality and cost management tools. The system is based on the premise that the process of rehabilitation reduces and/or compensates for a client's impairments and facilitates the reduction and compensation of functional limitations and disabilities. To ensure that a client progresses across these three phases of rehabilitation in the manner that is the most effective and efficient and ensures an outcome that is of value, the team must:

- Select from an array of potential outcomes the most appropriate one for the client.
- Develop and implement a client management plan that is tightly tied to that outcome.
- Develop and implement a process management plan that is driven by the preestablished expected outcome, monitors the client's progress toward that outcome throughout the course of rehabilitation, and

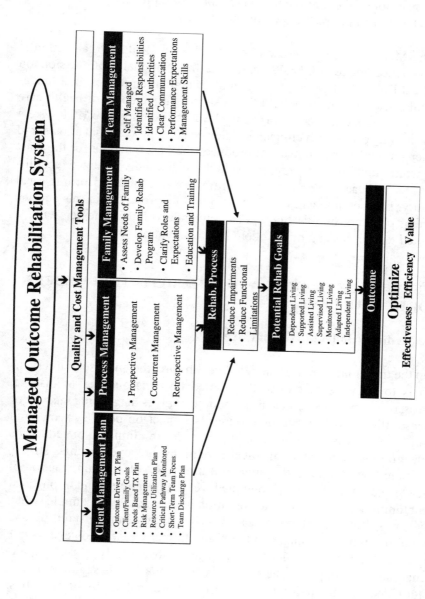

Figure 4–1 Managed Outcome Rehabilitation System

contributes to process improvement through individual and diagnostic group based outcome studies.
- Incorporate the family into the rehabilitation process.
- Develop and implement management skills.

The MORsystem is based on both the World Health Organization's[1] consequence model of health care and the National Commission on Medical Rehabilitation and Research's[2] rehabilitation model. In a fundamental sense, both models hold that a successful outcome of health care intervention is one that reduces a client's level of disability. The MORsystem provides the team with a clinical decision-making process that allows it to render services in a manner that produces the best outcome for the least cost while simultaneously preserving high-quality individualized rehabilitation as well as preserving one's professional ethics and professional identity. Each component of the system will be presented in this and the ensuing chapters of this book. The remainder of this chapter will be devoted to a discussion of the client management plan.

OVERVIEW OF MEDICAL AND REHABILITATION MODELS OF HEALTH CARE

The Medical Model of Health Care

In the traditional medical model of health care, the purpose of intervention is to alleviate or reduce the immediate consequences of disease, illness, or injury. The medical intervention involves diagnosing the type of disease, illness, or injury; identifying its impact on body systems; and treating the disease, illness, or injury in order to eliminate or reduce its impact on the body. Many medical conditions, however, such as stroke, traumatic brain injury, and spinal cord injury, set off a chain reaction of consequences that extend beyond the level of physiologic and/or physical symptom relief of a pathologic condition in the body. For example, when a person suffers a stroke, medical measures are taken to sustain life and control or minimize damage to the brain. In many cases, however, some degree of brain damage does occur, which subsequently causes impairments such as hemiplegia, hemianopsia, and aphasia. These impairments, in turn, decrease the individual's ability to perform daily living activities. Thus, the medical model of the intervention addresses the primary effects of a disease, illness, or injury but does not address their secondary and tertiary impacts.

In 1980, the World Health Organization (WHO) proposed a model of health care intervention that not only encompassed the level of pathology but also the consequences of that pathology.[3] This model (Exhibit 4–1), based on an earlier disablement model proposed by Nagi,[4] holds that the relief of symptoms alone is not the sole measure of a successful intervention outcome. It recognizes that a disease, illness, or injury not only impairs bodily structures and functions, but also reduces one's ability to meet daily living needs (e.g., personal, household, community, and work activities of daily living). Within the context of the WHO model, a more important measure of the success of health care intervention is the degree to which the consequences of the pathology are reduced.

The Rehabilitation Model of Health Care

More recently, the National Commission on Medical Rehabilitation and Research (NCMRR) developed a model of rehabilitation intervention,[5] which is based on the WHO and Nagi models but which extends them in a manner that reflects the purpose and focus of rehabilitation. According to this model (Exhibit 4–2), the scope of rehabilitation covers the domains of pathophysiology, impairment, functional limitation, disability, and societal limitation. An application of this model to speech-language pathology, occupational therapy, and physical therapy is shown in Exhibit 4–3.

Exhibit 4–1 World Health Organization's Consequence Model

Injury/Illness → *Impairment* → *Disability* → *Handicap*

- *Illness/Injury* (pathology): The interruption of, or interference with, normal structures (e.g., CVA, TBI, and SCI).
- *Impairment:* The loss and/or abnormality of cognitive, communicative, physical, emotional, physiological, or anatomical structure or function.
- *Disability:* Any restriction or lack of ability to perform an activity in the manner considered normal.
- *Handicap:* A disadvantage that limits or prevents the fulfillment of a role that is normal for that individual.

Exhibit 4–2 NCMRR Model of Rehabilitation

> *Pathophysiology* → *Impairment* → *Functional Limitation* →
> *Disability* → *Societal Limitation*
>
> - *Pathophysiology:* The interruption of, or interference with, normal physiological and developmental processes and structures (e.g., CVA, TBI, SCI, etc.).
> - *Impairment:* The loss or abnormality of cognitive, emotional or physiological function, or anatomical structure.
> - *Functional Limitation:* Any restriction or lack of ability to perform an action in the manner consistent with the purpose of an organ or organ system.
> - *Disability:* An inability or limitation in performing tasks, activities, and roles.
> - *Societal Limitation:* Restrictions caused by structural or attitudinal barriers that limit fulfillment of roles or deny access to services and opportunities.

The Rehabilitation Process

The purpose of rehabilitation, then, is not simply to decrease a client's level of impairment. The purpose is to increase a client's ability to perform usual and customary tasks, activities, and roles, and/or to gain the ability to perform new ones. The rehabilitation process is the provision of services that facilitates the client's progress toward the goals of impairment reduction and functional limitation and disability reduction.

Each phase of rehabilitation leads to a specific outcome that provides the basis to go forward to the next phase. The reduction of impairments leads to the outcome of increased ability to produce the isolated skills that are prerequisite to regaining the ability to perform daily living tasks (i.e., reduction of functional limitations). The reduction of functional limitations leads to the outcome of the ability to perform daily living tasks (i.e., disability reduction) and the resumption of roles in life that are meaningful to the client, the client's family, and society at large. Historically, when a client was admitted for rehabilitation, each discipline evaluated the client and established their own discipline-specific goals and treatment plan. While each discipline's goals and treatment plan guided its efforts, it did not provide a basis for a coordinated interdisciplinary approach. Today, a

Exhibit 4–3 NCMRR Model of Rehabilitation Applied to Specialities

---

Speech-Language Pathology

Pathophysiology: Left cerebrovascular accident (CVA) anterior branch of middle cerebral artery.

Impairment: The left CVA causes verbal apraxia (impairment).

Functional Limitation: The verbal apraxia (impairment), in turn, causes the client's inability to produce three to four word phrases (functional limitation).

Disability: The inability to produce three to four word phrases (functional limitation) results in the client's inability to communicate his health care needs to his doctor (disability).

Societal Limitation: Playing bridge was a favorite social activity that both the client and his wife enjoyed before his CVA. When they returned to this activity, the client used an assistive device to hold his cards, was clumsy in their manipulation, and he was unable to converse easily with the other players. After a short period of time, they found fewer and fewer invitations to play bridge and an increasing number of excuses from others to join them for bridge at their home.

Occupational Therapy

Pathophysiology: Left CVA anterior branch of middle cerebral artery.

Impairment: The left CVA causes right upper extremity weakness (impairment).

Functional Limitation: The right upper extremity weakness (impairment), in turn, causes the client's inability to grasp and hold small objects (functional limitation).

Disability: The inability to grasp and hold small objects results in the client's inability to feed himself independently (disability).

Societal Limitation: Dining out was a primary leisure activity of both the client and his wife prior to his CVA. When they tried eating out at a fast food restaurant, people stared at them and reflected negative facial expressions as she assisted him with his meal. They no longer go out for dinner.

Physical Therapy

Pathophysiology: Left CVA anterior branch of middle cerebral artery.

Impairment: The left CVA caused right lower extremity weakness (impairment).

---

continues

Exhibit 4–3 continued

Functional Limitation: The right lower extremity weakness (impairment),
    in turn, causes the client to have poor static standing balance (functional
    limitation).
Disability: The poor static standing balance (functional limitation) results
    in the client's inability to safely take a bath independently (disability).
Societal Limitation: The client requires a wheelchair for mobility and the
    bathroom doorway is not wide enough to allow access. The family does
    not have the money to modify the doorway.

team's ability to facilitate a client's movement through the three phases of
rehabilitation in the most effective and efficient manner is dependent upon
a tightly coordinated interdisciplinary team treatment effort. Everyone
must be going in the same direction, at the same time, and for the same
reason. Building a house has a certain rudimentary analogy to rehabilitation. First, one determines what they want the house to look like and how
it will function before construction begins (i.e., the outcome of the myriad
craftsmen's skills are specified before construction begins). Then a blueprint (client management plan) is drawn up that specifies where and how
each part of the house is to be built (i.e., the specification of which
craftsmen will be needed, as well as when, where, and how each is to
function). In rehabilitation, the client management plan specifies the
expected outcome of the rehabilitation team's interventions before rehabilitation begins and is also the blueprint that team members will need to
attain that outcome.

CLIENT MANAGEMENT PLAN

- Outcome-Driven Treatment Plan
- Client/Family Goals
- Needs-Based Treatment Planning
- Risk Management
- Resource Utilization Plan
- Critical Pathway Monitored
- Short-Term Team Focus
- Team Discharge Plan

OUTCOME-DRIVEN TREATMENT PLAN

The MORsystem is based on the service delivery principle that the first step in clinical case management is ensuring that all members of the rehabilitation team are treating toward a common client outcome goal—a goal against which all disciplines can measure progress toward their discipline-specific short-term goals.

In the MORsystem, the team selects the client outcome goal from the menu of possible outcomes provided by the Functional Living Scale (Exhibit 4–4). This scale is composed of eight functional living levels as shown in the Functional Living Level column. Its purpose is to identify a client's most probable lifestyle either at the end of a given phase of rehabilitation or when discharged from rehabilitation. For example, the outcome of "supported living" often represents the lifestyle that is re- quired to continue rehabilitation at home through a home health agency. The outcome of "assisted living" may allow the client to move into outpatient rehabilitation where his or her disabilities can be reduced to the degree that the expected outcome lifestyle will be that of "adapted living." In this context, one's lifestyle is defined as the least restrictive place of residence (Place of Residence column), the frequency and manner of accessing community resources (Community Access), the degree to which clients can manage their own health, safety, and welfare (Level of Super- vision column), the degree to which clients can perform their usual and customary daily living activities (Client's Level of Ability column), and the amount of assistance clients will need from another to perform their usual and customary daily living activities (Level of Assistance Required from Another column). The "total care" level of living on this scale is not an expected rehabilitation outcome. A client who holds an outcome of total care is not an appropriate rehabilitation candidate. In many cases, how- ever, a client may enter rehabilitation at the total care level of living with the expectation that the outcome will be a higher level of living.

Not all clients need the same type of assistance; consequently, the team indicates whether the required assistance will be physical, cognitive, communicative, perceptual, emotional, and/or social. In the "place of residence" column, it will be noted that "own home" and "family member home" are shown for dependent through monitored living levels. These places of residence are feasible only to the degree that the family is physically, emotionally, and/or logistically (in terms of work and child

Exhibit 4–4 Functional Living Scale

Name: _____

Date: _____

Prior Functional Level ____   Expected Functional Level ____

Current Functional Level ____   Achieved Functional Level ____

Functional Living level	Place of Residence	Community Access	Level of Supervision	Client's Level of Ability	Level of Assistance Required From Another
Independent Living	• Own Home • Retirement Facility • Family Member Home	Daily to perform all usual and customary community activities. Can drive.	None.	Independent in all usual & customary daily living skills	None other than that degree of assistance that normally occurs in the course of cooperative daily living.
Adapted Living	• Own Home • Retirement Facility • Family Member Home	Daily to perform all usual and customary community activities. Can drive, may require car modifications, use public transportation - may require modifications to access.	None.	Mod. independent in all usual & customary daily living skills with: Modified environment — Assistive devices/equipment — Compensatory strategies — More than usual amount of time — ① Directs others to meet needs —	None other than that degree of assistance that normally occurs in the course of cooperative daily living.
Monitored Living	• Own Home • Family Member Home • Board & Care Facility	Daily to perform all usual and customary community activities. Can drive/or use public transportation or obtain it from another.	As needed advice regarding general health, safety and welfare when requested by client.	Performs all usual & customary daily living skills with as needed assistance requested by client.	As needed assistance: Physical — Cognitive — Communicative —
Supervised Living	• Own Home • Family Member Home • Board and Care Facility	2-3Xwk. to shop for needs, access health care, personal care, leisure activity. Cannot drive. Can use public transportation or obtain it from another.	As needed initiated by another by phone, fax or in person to assure general health, safety and welfare.	Performs at least 90% of all usual & customary daily living skills.	10% or less assistance: Physical — Cognitive — Communicative —
Assisted Living	• Own Home • Family Member Home • Assisted Living Facility	1-2Xwk. to shop for needs, access health care, personal care or leisure activities. Cannot drive. Can use public transportation or obtain it from another with assist.	Direct supervision every 8 hrs. during waking hours to assure general health, safety and welfare.	Performs 75% or more of a reduced type and amount of usual & customary daily living skills.	25% or less assistance: Physical — Cognitive — Communicative —
Supported Living	• Own Home • Family Member Home • Extended Care Facility	2-3X/mo. for personal care, access health care or leisure activities. Private transportation only. May need to be modified transportation	Direct supervision every 3 hrs. during waking hours and as needed overnight monitoring to assure general health, safety and welfare.	Performs 50%-75% of personal care and a reduced type and amount of household management, community access & leisure skills.	25% to 50% assistance: Physical — Cognitive — Communicative —

continues

Exhibit 4–4 continued

Dependent Living	• Own Home • Family Member Home • Extended Care Facility	1Xmo. for health care need. Modified transportation only.	Supervising person always present. Client checked no more than every hour during day and scheduled night time checks to assure general health, safety and welfare.	Performs at least 25% of personal care and leisure skills.	75% assistance: Physical — Cognitive — Communicative —
Total Care	• Own Home • Family Member Home • SNF	None	Supervising person always present. Client checked no less than every 30 minutes.	Performs less than 25% of personal care.	100% assistance: Physical — Cognitive — Communicative —

care schedules) able to provide the amount of supervision and assistance required for each level, or if the client/family have the financial resources to pay a caregiver to provide the required supervision and assistance.

Traditionally, the expected outcome has been determined solely on the basis of the type and severity of a client's impairments, functional limitations, and disabilities. In today's health care delivery system, the team must select an outcome on the basis of the following factors:

- level of care
- payment
- customer preference
- type and severity of impairments, functional limitations, and disabilities

Levels of Care

In the early era of rehabilitation, a client's total course of rehabilitation was provided solely at the inpatient level of care. As such, the expected outcome that the rehabilitaiton team selected was one that could be attained by the time of discharge from rehabilitation. Today, as noted in Chapter 3, there exists a multilevel menu of rehabilitation options. Depending upon client need, rehabilitation can be obtained in an inpatient acute rehabilitation program, a skilled nursing facility, a subacute rehabilitation unit, or at home through a home health agency, as well as through a wide array of outpatient programs. Each of these care options has a different level of associated cost. Payers want rehabilitation to be provided at the most medically appropriate and least expensive level of care at any given point. As a result, a client's progress through the three phases of rehabilitation will usually span several levels of care rather than one. Consequently, the team must select the client outcome goal that best matches the admission criteria of the next level of care to which the client will be discharged rather than the ultimate outcome that their clinical assessments indicate.

Payment

A client may have the potential for the outcome of adapted living but has a health insurance policy that will only pay for the services needed to produce an outcome of supervised living. In this instance, the team must treat toward the supervised living outcome. Variations in what and how much health care plans cover will often lead to the determination of outcome on the basis of coverage rather than clinical parameters. This creates a difficult situation for the team, the client, and the client's family. It is entirely possible that, on any given day, the team could evaluate several patients and determine that all have the same diagnosis, type and severity of impairments and disabilities, and the same prognosis. The team must select different outcomes for each, however, because of differences in the health care coverage for each client or the client's family. The team potentially could believe it's been placed in an ethically compromising position and the clients and their families could feel unfairly treated. Here, the case manager plays a key role in either preventing, or at least minimizing, a negative reaction by all parties. The case manager must inform the team of any coverage limitations before the assessment begins so that it can begin shaping clinical decisions prior to the initial team conference. It is extremely important that the team members bear in mind that the client's health insurance coverage is out of their control and that they are functioning ethically within the constraints imposed upon them. The case manager must also review any coverage limitations with the client/family during the evaluation process to help them understand how and why their policy may place constraints on what the team will be able to accomplish. It is the responsibility of the team to identify any community resources that may help the client continue to progress after discharge and to build them into the client's discharge plan.

Customer Preference

The rehabilitation team may find that it must select an outcome based on the customer's perceived needs. For example, a client and/or family may desire an outcome that is the equivalent of supervised living when the client holds the potential for adapted living. When faced with such a circumstance, the team must treat toward the outcome that the client and/or family is motivated to work toward. To treat toward the higher level outcome may produce positive results within the context of a structured rehabilitation program, but the outcome will not be maintained after the discharge because the client and/or family will not take the necessary measures to support it.

Case Study

Prior to her stroke, BT was a homemaker. She had devoted her entire life toward managing the home and raising four children. Three of her children were married and living nearby; the fourth lived at home. She was very active in her church and participated in activities with a tightly knit extended family. After her stroke, her husband and children took the position, which was typical and expected in their culture, that they were now responsible for her care. In essence, they retired her from her homemaker job. While BT held the prognosis of adapted living, the team, client, and family agreed upon the outcome of assisted living.

* * * * *

Type and Severity of Impairments, Functional Limitations, and Disabilities

A client and/or family may desire an outcome of independent living and may have the financial resources to support the intense rehabilitation program required to achieve such an outcome. The nature and severity of the client's impairments and disabilities, however, will only support the outcome of supervised living. In this scenario, the team must treat toward the clinically dictated outcome and work with the client and family to help them understand why their desired outcome cannot be realized.

How To Select the Client's Expected Outcome

The client outcome selected by the team must meet the following criteria. It must be:

- relevant (The achieved abilities must be functional in the discharge environment.)
- utilitarian (The achieved abilities must be the most practical way of meeting daily living needs.)
- efficient (The achieved abilities must be performed at the rate of speed and degree of consistency that meet the demands of the discharge environment and must be performed in a manner that requires the least effort for the client and caregiver.)

In the case of managed care clients, the team selects the expected outcome on the basis of the following parameters:

- the client's prior level of living (One's prior level of living is the level on the Functional Living Scale that best describes the level at which the client performed his or her daily living skills prior to the debilitating medical episode. It is extremely important to clearly establish a client's prior level of functioning. Not all clients will be at the independent level of living prior to their medical episode and the selection of an outcome that is higher than their premorbid level of functioning must be avoided.)
- the client's current level of living (The client's current level of living is the level on the Functional Living Scale that best describes the level at which the client performs his or her usual and customary daily living skills at the time of the rehabilitation evaluation.)
- the length of treatment authorized by the payer
- the disciplines that the payer has authorized to treat the client
- the frequency and intensity of treatment for each discipline the payer has authorized
- the level of living that meets the admission criteria of the next level of care
- the outcome that best fits the level of daily living skills that the client wants to perform
- the outcome that best fits the level of daily living skills the family will allow the client to perform
- the outcome that best fits the family's physical, logistical, emotional, and/or financial capabilities to support it
- the extent to which the client's impairments and disabilities can be expected to be reduced

In the case of non–managed care clients, the team uses the following criteria to select the projected client outcome:

- the client's prior level of living (as described above)
- the client's current level of living (as described above)
- the outcome level that meets either the admission criteria of the next level of care or criteria for discharge from rehabilitation

- the outcome that best fits the level of daily living skills the client wants to perform
- the outcome that best fits the level of daily living skills the family will allow the client to perform
- the outcome that best fits the family's physical, logistical, emotional, and/or financial capabilities to support it
- the outcome that best fits the degree to which the client's impairments, functional limitations, and disabilities can be expected to be reduced.

CLIENT/FAMILY GOALS

Success in today's health care delivery system requires a fundamental shift in the therapist's perception, attitudes, and beliefs regarding the client's role and responsibilities. Therapists can no longer view clients as passive recipients of the therapist's knowledge and expertise. Active and informed participation of the client and family will be required to attain the best outcome in the shortest amount of time. Client and family involvement is also critical to an outcome that is satisfactory to both client and family and, therefore, sustained after discharge. To this end, therapists must facilitate their clients to become active decision-making partners. When clients are actively involved in establishing their own goals, they are more likely to have interest in and work toward them.[6] In the past, clients were encouraged to believe that the "locus of control" resided within the trained health professional. Either overtly or covertly, the professionals reinforced the clients' belief that only the therapist had the knowledge, skills, and judgment necessary to cure their problem. Clients were allowed to believe that therapists and events external to themselves would meet their needs and that they had no personal responsibility for, nor influence on, the outcome of the services they were provided. To be successful today, therapists must help their clients develop an "internal locus of control"— a belief that they can and must influence their own outcomes.[7,8] It has been shown that there is a positive relationship between internal locus of control and involvement, good coping skills, and emotional adaptation. All three of these factors are needed during the course of rehabilitation both to achieve the projected outcome as well as to sustain or enhance it after discharge. Failure to establish an internal locus of control creates the breeding ground for *learned helplessness. Learned helplessness* is a state of passivity and unwillingness to attempt problem solutions. It occurs when one repeatedly experiences failure in an attempt to control one's environment.[9] Clearly, learned helplessness is the antithesis of the goal of rehabilitation. Its presence prolongs rehabilitation and results in regression after discharge, two situations that are very expensive from both a quality of life and fiscal perspectives.

Identifying client and family goals is the first step in facilitating an internal locus of control. Knowledge of their goals allows the team to individualize the level of living goal that it selects for the client. When the expected level of living goal is individualized, a number of things occur that are fundamental to providing an outcome that has value:

- The client and/or family feels the team is responsive to them as an individual.
- Clients see the relationship between what they want and expect and the therapist's treatment goals and procedures.
- The clients take responsibility for the outcome and become active rather than passive participants in the rehabilitation process.
- When clients take their share of the responsibility for rehabilitation, a meaningful, utilitarian, and durable outcome is achieved.
- When all of the above occur, the expected outcome will be achieved at or before the expected time and, as a result, the customers (i.e., client, family, and payer) will be satisfied.

Goal Setting

Client/family goals are identified in the initial meeting between the client and the case manager. The degree to which the client can actively participate in goal setting depends upon where he or she falls on the Functional Living Scale. Active participation increases commensurately as one ascends the levels of living scale. To facilitate a sense of an internal locus of control, the case manager must first prepare the client/family to participate in goal setting. They enter this process as novices. Accordingly, the case manager must provide them with the information they will need to make informed decisions. To do this, the case manager describes and discusses the following aspects of rehabilitation and services:

The Rehabilitation Process. The case manager describes the three phases of rehabilitation and the various levels of care that the client may be admitted to when progressing across these phases of rehabilitation. The case manager also discusses the manner in which prognosis and/or funding will determine whether the client and family should anticipate involvement in one or all three of the phases.

The Purpose of Rehabilitation. The case manager educates the client and family about the purpose of rehabilitation and discusses the fact that rehabilitation functions to reduce and/or compensate for impairments, functional limitations, and disabilities but does not "cure" them. Additionally, the case manager presents the concept of *medical necessity*—the fact that the rehabilitation team can only justify continued treatment as long as the client is making significant practical improvement. *Significant practical improvement* is defined to them as impairment reduction that results in the measurable reduction of functional limitations and the continued reduction in functional limitations that results in measurable disability reduction. The client's and family's understanding of the purpose of rehabilitation is absolutely essential to the process of helping them establish an internal locus of control. In most instances, their perceptions, attitudes, and beliefs related to health care are based on medical problems that have taken them to a physician's office or hospital for acute medical care. From this experience they develop the health care concept of: "When I get sick, I see a physician, the physician gives me medicine and I get better." Thus, when most clients and their families enter rehabilitation they naturally bring this—their only health care paradigm—with them. An external locus of control focuses on the impairments as the problem and the "doctor" (therapists) who will cure them. Clients and families fail to understand that the purpose of rehabilitation is not curing impairments but rather reducing functional limitations and disabilities through compensatory techniques, devices, and equipment. Their focus on impairments alone typically results in their failure to support and reinforce compensatory strategies because they believe they will not be needed when the impairments are "cured" by the therapists. As can be anticipated, their external locus of control paradigm rapidly leads to frustration, anger, and disappointment as they see a chronic degree of impairment remain and the team, from their perspective, that is ignoring the "real problems."

Covered Services. The case manager identifies and discusses the type, frequency, and duration of services that can be provided within the scope of their health care funding.

Purpose of Covered Services. The case manager provides a general description of the therapy techniques that will be provided by each of the covered disciplines.

Client/Family Request for Services

After this information has been presented, discussed, and clarified, the case manager and the client/family mutually explore their concerns and goals. First, the case manager asks them to describe the problems (impairments) that they want the team to address in its treatment plan. Once a problem list has been developed, the case manager asks the client/family to identify the specific disabilities that they believe must be reduced in order to function successfully in his or her discharge place of residence. The Client/Family Request for Services questionnaire (Appendix 4–A) is a useful tool to help the client and family identify the disabilities they believe are the most important. This questionnaire is sent out to the family before the client is admitted. Typically, the case manager uses the responses from the questionnaire in the meeting with the client and family to individualize the list of disabilities as much as possible. To this end, the case manager should emphasize that it is important to identify both the client's usual and customary daily living activities and the degree to which they believe they will be required in his or her discharge place of residence. If a questionnaire such as this is not used or, as sometimes happens, is not filled out, the case manager then poses questions such as, "What would you most like to be able to do at home, work, in the community, or with friends when you are discharged from this program?" or " What must you absolutely be able to do in order to live at home and enjoy life again?" After establishing the problem and disability lists, the next step is to request that they prioritize each list according to what they believe are the first, second, third, etc. most important impairments and disabilities that they would like the team to address. This prioritization process is important. First, it begins the process of facilitating an internal locus of control. Second, it focuses treatment on what the customer wants and, finally, if treatment authorization is limited, it helps the team to focus quickly on what is most important to the customer in the limited amount of time available. In essence, prioritizing in this context is asking the client and family how they want to spend their money. It is also important to know their priorities in order to sequence treatment in a manner that is consistent with their expectations. Since a client's/family's functional status, knowledge, perceptions, and priorities change across time, it is important to review and modify their goals during the course of rehabilitation.

Treatment should always be directed toward the client/family goals unless their goals either cannot be attained at all, cannot be attained at their current level of care, and/or cannot be attained within the constraints imposed by the payer. Further, the team must always add any goals left out by the client or family whose absence would place the client at risk for additional injury/illness and/or secondary complications. The team also adds goals they believe complement or extend the client/family goals. Finally, goals not identified by the client/family, but which, in the opinion of the team, are important to the client's rehabilitation success, are discussed with the client/family following the initial client conference in order to clarify their rationale.

Case Study

RN, who had a right cerebrovascular accident (CVA), was admitted for acute inpatient rehabilitation with an expected outcome of monitored living. He and his wife said they would like to be able to do two things after discharge from inpatient rehabilitation that were most important to them prior to his stroke: (1) dine out in restaurants, and (2) travel. The team, client, and his wife identified several functional limitations that would result in particular disabilities while dining out or traveling. The client could not spontaneously find his eating utensils or find all of the food on his plate, he spilled food on the table and on himself, and he knocked over items on the table.

If traveling with his wife on public transportation, he could be at risk for falls because he couldn't accurately judge the distance between himself and others or environmental barriers, couldn't accurately identify curbs and steps or judge their height, and he couldn't find his way from his room to the therapy areas and back.

The team established the following goals to address these functional limitations and, thereby, reduce his disabilities. Within three weeks, the client would require standby assistance to:

1. self-cue for position sense to maintain appropriate sitting and standing posture
2. self-cue for proper walking speed
3. self-cue for proper walking balance

4. self-cue for visual and auditory attention to environment
5. self-cue for visual scanning of environment, objects in the environment, and tasks
6. self-cue for judgment of distances (e.g., distance between self and environmental barrier, distance between hand and eating utensils)
7. self-cue for planning sequence of motor movement events needed to navigate environmental barriers and handle objects
8. self-cue for path finding
9. self-cue to monitor effectiveness of his solution to problems encountered in working the the tasks envolved in goals 1–8 and to implement alternative solutions if needed

Each discipline established specific goals related to each of these team goals. Treatment was first carried out in the context of simulated activities in the therapy areas and then in real-life situations similar to those encountered while dining out and accessing public transportation. RN achieved these goals by the end of three weeks and he and his wife were able to resume their previous activities.

NEEDS-BASED TREATMENT PLANNING

Once the expected outcome and client/family goals have been established, the team, client, and/or family must next identify the disabilities that must be reduced in order to attain the expected outcome—they must determine exactly what abilities the client will need to master in order to support the expected outcome. Nagi defines disability as a limitation in performing one's roles within one's natural sociocultural environments (e.g., the roles of homemaker, worker, husband, wife, father, mother, or volunteer).[10] The presence and degree of disability are determined and defined by the degree to which there is a discrepancy between a person's unique "status indicators" (the person's potential role[s] in the environment) and their "activity indicators" (the activities that the person must be able to perform within that environment). According to Brown, a person has a disability only to the extent that they are unable to perform the activities that will be required to fulfill the roles expected in their particular sociocultural environment.[11] Within this context, disability is determined by the relationship between an individual's expected roles, activities required to carry out those roles, task performance capacities to carry out the activities, and the environmental conditions within which the person's roles and capacities will be performed.

Case Studies

Mrs. D, post-CVA, held a monitored living outcome—it was expected that she would return to her own home with monitoring provided as needed by her grown children, who lived close to her. Her goals included the reduction of disabilities related to meal preparation, housekeeping, and laundry. Two weeks into her rehabilitation, Mrs. D decided that she would rather live in a retirement facility that provided services such as meals, room cleaning, and laundry. Because Mrs. D would not be required to prepare meals, keep house, and do laundry in this environment, they were no longer areas of disabilities, and consequently, treatment related to these goals was discontinued. Mrs. D, however, would not have assistance in getting from one location to another in the retirement home and on outings, nor would she be supervised in taking her medications. Further, while she would not need to do her own laundry, she would have to be able to sort her clothes in accordance to hot and cold wash and dry cleaning. She also would still be called upon to communicate in social situations. Accordingly, the goals related to path finding, medication management, and appropriate communication pragmatics were continued and the laundry goal was modified to focus on sorting her clothes because these remained disabilities within the context of this new living environment.

* * * * *

RL and FC each experienced a right hemisphere stroke. Both had similar impairments of left hemiplegia, hemisensory neglect, and visual neglect. RL was employed and one year from retirement when he had his stroke and FC was 57 years old and employed when she had hers. Both had the expected outcome of adapted living, including return to work. RL decided to take the early retirement offered to him and FC wanted to return to the modified job that had been offered to her. RL's previous roles had been sole financial provider for his family; friend, companion, and lover for his wife; and the planner and implementor of fishing trips and gambling trips to the local casino. His wife had the role of managing all of the household activities of daily living.

FC was unmarried and without children. Her previous roles had been that of worker, friend, and companion to people at work and manager of all household activities of daily living. As might be expected, the type and nature of the gap between RL's and FC's expected roles, the activities required to carry them out, and the degree of environmental support available to carry them out were very different. For RL, the gap existed solely in the area of accessing his and his wife's leisure activities. For FC, on the other hand, the gap existed in the areas of work, household management, and accessing leisure activities. As a consequence, the team focused only on those disabilities that created barriers to leisure activities for RL and on work, household management, and leisure activities for FC.

*   *   *   *   *

Thus, while impairments and functional limitations create potentially disabling conditions, a disability is not actually the consequence of them. A disability is not in the person per se nor is it in the person's environment. It is the degree to which a gap exists between a person's capabilities and expected roles, the activities required to support those roles, and the degree to which the environment does not compensate for the person's impairments and functional limitations.[12] If a gap does not exist, then neither does a disability. A gap may occur at a later date, however, if there is a decline in a client's performance capabilities and/or degree of environmental support. If and when this occurs, the client at that moment becomes a candidate for a reevaluation to determine whether disabilities now exist that are barriers to meeting daily living needs.

The team uses needs-based treatment planning to develop a client treatment plan that meets the following criteria:

1. It must be based on the environment(s) within which the client will be expected to function and the roles expected of the client in those environments.
2. It must only focus on those impairments, functional limitations, and disabilities that create a gap between the client's capabilities and the demands of the environment. As noted earlier, it may be appropriate to focus on other impairments, functional limitations, and disabilities if and when environmental demands change.
3. It must be tightly focused on only those specific activities that the client must be able to perform in the environment in order to carry out his or her role(s).

Needs-based treatment planning (Exhibit 4–5) is based on the following clinical reasoning process:

Exhibit 4–5 Needs-Based Treatment Planning

Environments	→	Roles	→	Capabilities	→	Supports	→	Impairments
Home		Wife		Safety		Physical		Physiologic
		Husband		Personal ADL		Cognitive		Skeletal
Community		Mother		Household ADL		Communicative		Physical
		Father		Community		Emotional		Perceptual
Work/School		Daughter		Work/Education		Social		Cognitive
		Son		Sexuality		Financial		Emotional
Leisure		Worker		Social Interaction		Transportation		Behavioral
		Homemaker		Self-Development		Leisure		
		Sister		Spirituality				
		Brother		Etc.				
		Leader						
		Supporter						
		Friend						
		Lover						
		Mediator						
		Etc.						

Note: ADL = activities of daily living

- Given the client's projected outcome, within what functional domains (or environments) will the client be able to function?
- Given those functional domains, what role(s) will the client be expected to carry out?
- Given those functional domains and roles, what capabilities will be required to carry out the roles in those domains?
- Given those functional domains, roles, and required capabilities, what supports will the environment be able to provide to assist in carrying them out?
- Given the required abilities, what specific impairments and/or functional limitations must be reduced to facilitate the performance of those abilities at the level required to fill the gap between the client's current level of function and the demands of the environment in order to carry out his or her roles?

Identifying Disabilities

The identification of disabilities individualizes the expected outcome the team has selected from the Functional Living Scale. The disabilities that are identified by the previous clinical decision-making process define the specific abilities in the client's Level of Ability column in the Functional Living Scale that the given client must achieve in order to function at any given level of living.

Using the information derived from these questions, the team then uses the following set of questions to determine whether there is a gap between any performance ability that will be required in the place of discharge, the demands of that environment, and the degree of support available:

- What usual and customary personal, household, community, work/educational, and/or leisure daily living activities did the client carry out before the illness/injury?
- What usual and customary personal, household, community, work/educational, and/or leisure daily living activity skills will be required for the client to function in his or her place of discharge?
- What usual and customary personal, household, community, work/educational, and/or leisure daily living activities does the client want to carry out?

- What usual and customary personal, household, community, work/ educational, and/or leisure daily living activities does the family want the client to be able to perform?

- What, if any, unusual and noncustomary personal, household, community, work/educational, and leisure activities of daily living (ADLs) will be required of the client to function in the discharge environment?

- What usual and customary and/or unusual personal, household, community, work/educational, and/or leisure daily living activity skills will the client be able to perform and at what level?

The team can organize and preserve the information derived from these questions on the Individual Daily Living Skills checklist (Exhibit 4–6). This is a non–discipline-specific checklist. All performance domains are dependent in some way upon perceptual, physical, cognitive, communicative, and emotional skills. Consequently, as noted in the checklist, all disciplines involved in a client's treatment plan are expected to write short-term goals related to the areas of disability identified by the client, family, and team.

The performance domains and the abilities within each of them are those that are most frequently identified in the general rehabilitation population, but may not represent all possible types of disabilities. For this reason, the category of other is included in each of the performance domains so that abilities unique to a given client may be added.

As clients move from one level of care to another and from one phase of rehabilitation to another, they usually move from a focus on safety and personal care performance domains to the broader domains of daily living skills. Most typically, the subacute level of rehabilitation focuses primarily on the personal care performance. The inpatient acute level of care also focuses on this area and may also begin to address some of the safety, health maintenance, and household management performance domains. The home health level of care may address any remaining personal care disabilities, as well as disabilities in the safety, health maintenance, household management, community access (depending upon payer), and leisure performance domains. At the outpatient rehabilitation level of care, some personal care issues may remain, but the primary focus is usually on

Exhibit 4-6 Individual Daily Living Skills

Name: _____
MR#: _____

Safety	Date:	% EFFORT EXPENDED		
Seek help				
Handle emergencies				
Recognize safety hazards or dangerous conditions and take appropriate action to be safe.				
Health Maintenance				
Medication management				
Maintain proper exercise				
Follow proper diet				
Seek and obtain routine health care services				
Recognize signs of illness/injury and take appropriate action				
Cope with stress				
Personal Care				
Bathing				
Dressing				
Grooming / Hygiene				
Feeding				

Household Management	Date:	% EFFORT EXPENDED		
Clothing care				
Housekeeping				
Meal preparation				
House maintenance				
Financial management				
Time management				
Cooperative living				
Child care				
Community Access				
Shopping for needs and running errands				
Money management				
Access and utilize public resources				
Transportation				
Cooperative social interaction				
Productive Activity				
Paid productive activity				
Non-paid volunteer activity				
Leisure				
Solo leisure activities				
Attend spectator events				
Participate in games with others				
Participate in social activities				

% Effort Expended by Client

Complete Independence	100%
Modified Independent 100% — requires extra time, compensatory strategies	
Supervision	94% – 99%
Minimal Assist	75% – 94%
Moderate Assist	50% – 74%
Maximal Assist	25% – 49%
Total Assist	less than 25%

Instructions: (1) Enter date of initial evaluation. (2) Enter client's ability to perform (% effort expended) each of his/her usual and customary daily living skills in the column below the date. (3) Enter date of next progress reports thereafter and the client's ability to perform each of his/her usual and customary daily living skills in column under each date.

safety, health maintenance, household management, community access, productive activity, and leisure disabilities that are usual and customary for the client or will be new abilities required to meet environmental demands.

Selecting Impairments/Functional Limitations

After the team has identified a client's disabilities, it must further individualize the treatment plan by identifying the impairments and functional limitations that must absolutely be improved in order to reduce the client's disabilities. To this end, the following decision-making criteria are used:

- Which impairments/functional limitations are directly related to and causing a disability?
- Of those impairments/functional limitations, which require the knowledge, skills, and judgment of a therapist to help the client learn the skills required to carry out the activities that meet the demands of the client's environment?
- Of those impairments/functional limitations, which hold the greatest potential to improve?

RISK MANAGEMENT

Impairments and their resultant disabilities are directly caused by a medical condition such as a stroke, spinal cord injury, or limb amputation. The degree to which rehabilitation can reduce these results of pathology, however, is related to two factors: (1) the severity of the impairments and disabilities that are directly attributable to the medical condition, and (2) the presence of pre- and/or postmorbid conditions and risk factors that are either potential barriers to the attainment of the projected outcome or hold the potential to cause regression from that outcome after discharge. Historically, therapists have focused their assessment and treatment skills solely on the client's impairments, functional limitations, and disabilities. Today, they must broaden their scope of responsibilities to include risk identification, risk management, and risk prevention. Risk management, therefore, is a dynamic and ongoing clinical decision-making process that is the responsibility of the entire team.

It results in increased effectiveness of ongoing client treatment, sustained client progress during the course of rehabilitation, the client's attainment of the outcome goal at or before the expected date of discharge, and the maintenance or enhancement of the client's outcome level of living after discharge from rehabilitation.

To produce these results, risk management must be both proactive (anticipate and plan for potential client risk) and immediately reactive (immediately initiate a planned response to a risk that has occurred). Both proactive and reactive risk management are based on the following procedures:

- identification of type and degree of client risk
- identification of causal factors
- establishment of measurable and time-framed risk management goals
- continuous monitoring of progress toward the risk management goals in client conferences

Categories of Risk

Risk factors fall into the categories of premorbid conditions, secondary conditions, response to disablement, and environmental factors.[13]

Premorbid Conditions. These include preexisting medical conditions, such as diabetes or chronic obstructive pulmonary disease; lifestyle behaviors, such as alcohol and substance abuse; attitudes such as unhealthy nutritional habits; and environmental influences, such as dysfunctional family relationships or the lack of a support system.

Secondary Conditions. These include conditions that occur as a result of a primary impairment, such as pressure sores, contractions, urinary tract infections, and depression.

Response to Disablement. These are conditions that occur as a result of the client's reaction to being disabled, such as reduced activity level due to fear of falling, use of alcohol, anger, or denial.

Environmental Factors. These include the need for structural modifications at home/work/school, access to public buildings and public transportation, and access to health care, as well as employer/societal attitudes toward disabled persons.

Client assessment should not only include identification of the client's type and severity of impairments and disabilities, but also include a determination of whether risk factors exist. The type, amount, and severity of risk factors should be considered by the team when it establishes the expected outcome. It is possible that a client may have the potential for a certain outcome from the standpoint of the type or severity of his or her impairments and disabilities but a lower outcome when risk factors are taken into consideration. Once the team identifies the existence of risk factors, it develops goals and treatment approaches to address them. The goals typically become part of the Short-Term Team Focus and Discharge Plan sections of the client's treatment plan. Progress toward those goals are discussed and monitored at client conferences in the same manner that progress toward impairment and disability goals are monitored.

Case Studies

Premorbid Condition

RZ suffered a left CVA, which resulted in moderate right hemiplegia and mild aphasia. Prior to and after the CVA, she had arthritis, was obese, hypertensive, low in endurance secondary to excess weight, and had decreased pulmonary function. She also was depressed, had chronically smoked two packs of cigarettes a day, and was noncompliant with her arthritis, hypertension, and depression medications. Not only did these risk factors present barriers to rehabilitation, but they also placed RZ at a significant risk for another CVA.

Risk Management Plan. The team placed the medication noncompliance in the Short-Term Team Focus with the goal of compliance and independence in self-medication in two weeks. All team members were to discuss with her the purpose of each of her medications and the positive impact that appropriate self-medication would have on her recovery, as well as her general physical and emotional health. Speech pathology was responsible for developing and implementing a self-medication system and cueing strategy, which all team members reinforced by discussing it with the client in each of their respective treatment sessions during the course of rehabilitation. The team addressed the obesity and smoking risk factors in the discharge plan. The obesity goal was for the client to demonstrate knowledge of and implement a weight management plan by the time of discharge. To accomplish this, the dietitian, in consultation with the client, established an agreed-upon daily calorie intake. The dietitian also provided the client with a list of appropriate foods. Occupational therapy established goals related to meal planning, shopping, and meal preparation that were related to the required calorie intake and types of foods. Physical therapy developed and trained the client in a weight management exercise program that centered around low-impact activities such as walking and stair climbing. The exercise program was designed around her impairments to ensure that it was something she could easily continue after discharge. The physical therapist also facilitated the client's knowledge of and contact with a "mall walking" program and community aquatics program for people with arthritis by the time of discharge. Speech pathology incorporated all of the vocabulary related to the client's nutrition and weight management physical exercise program into the client's language rehabilitation program. Occupational therapy was also responsible for providing stroke prevention information and establishing discharge goals related to the ability to recognize the signs and symptoms of a stroke and the appropriate action to take. Social work focused on the interaction among all the risk factors as they related to the client's mental health and provided possible coping strategies. The social worker also explored the feasibility of smoking cessation and facilitated the client's knowledge of and contact with a cessation program prior to discharge.

* * * * *

Secondary Condition

CV incurred a right CVA with residual left hemiplegia, mild unawareness of impairments, and minimal left hemisensory neglect. She presented with a risk for a skin breakdown on the ventral surface of her left hand because of severe hypertonicity and impaired ability to adhere to splint-wearing schedule due to unawareness of impairment and left hemisensory neglect.

Risk Management Plan. Occupational therapy provided the client, the team, and the client's husband with the neurophysiologic rationale for the use of the splint and the potential consequences if it is not worn appropriately for the specified duration. Occupational therapy also provided the splinting schedule, and developed and implemented a self-cueing system to help CV compensate for her unawareness of impairment and hemisensory neglect. Speech pathology incorporated the splinting rationale, schedule, and self-cueing system into their treatment goals relating to judgment and problem solving. Physical therapy reinforced the rationale and importance of splinting and the self-cueing system in all of its treatment sessions. They also took measures to facilitate CV's understanding of how proper upper extremity movement related to her concerns about balance and mobility. All therapy disciplines reinforced the importance of the risk management plan and ensured that the client's husband understood it and would be responsible for assisting his wife with it every day.

* * * * *

Response to Disablement

RD, a 19-year-old man, sustained a T5-6 spinal cord injury as a result of a motorcycle accident. Prior to the accident, he lived in his own apartment and worked in his father's construction business. The client described himself as being very outgoing and into sports, loved working with his father, and loved the physical nature of construction work. Following the accident, RD and his family were emotionally devastated. The client was significantly depressed with suicidal thoughts and his father talked of having lost his "best friend." After a brief period of inpatient rehabilitation, RD was discharged to his parents' home and entered outpatient rehabilitation. It quickly became apparent that RD's mother and father were overhelping him. His father was lifting him for all transfers rather than allowing him to work on tasks that he and his parents were being taught in physical therapy. His father stated that he knew he shouldn't do what he was doing but that he couldn't help himself because he couldn't stand to see his son struggle. A similar situation was occurring with his mother with respect to dressing and catheter care.

The client encouraged the overhelping even though he expressed to his therapists his desire to be more independent. Clearly RD's and his family's response to the medical condition and its sequalae posed a major risk for successfully achieving the expected outcome of adapted living.

Risk Management Plan. The team established a Short-Term Focus of crisis counseling for RD's parents, concentrating on the long-term consequences of overhelping both for them and RD. The physical therapist negotiated an agreement from RD to engage in peer counseling with a person with the same level injury and to attend a spinal cord injury support group. Social work counseling focused on the dynamics of his allowing the overhelping.

* * * * *

Environmental Factors

FC had a right parietal CVA with residual mild left lower-extremity weakness, severe left upper-extremity weakness, moderate left visual neglect, and moderate left hemisensory neglect. In addition to her neurologically based depression, she was also significantly clinically depressed. FC was unmarried and without children or relatives in the immediate area. She stated that her work as a bank teller and her friends at work, with whom she enjoyed numerous after-work community activities, were "my life." If she could not return to work, FC was at a significant risk of regression from her expected discharge level of living skills, because without work, she would lose both her major life role as well as access to her social life. Given this, it was highly probable that her clinical depression would deepen and, consequently, make it more difficult to cope with her neurologically driven depression, both of which would cause her to withdraw from an active lifestyle. FC held the expected outcome of adapted living, which in her instance included return to work in some capacity.

Risk Management Plan. FC, together with her employer and the team, determined that she could not return to her usual and customary job as a bank teller but that she would be able to return to a customer relations position. Work requirements and workspace modifications relative to her inability to functionally use her left upper extremity, her left visual neglect, and left hemisensory neglect were identified by the team. The employer arranged a modified work schedule and the appropriate public transportation schedule and route were identified. A simulated workstation was developed in a clerical area of the rehabilitation hospital and all disciplines carried out their treatment in that environment. During this time, FC learned to use public transportation to travel to the hospital rather than the hospital van. Concurrently, FC attended group therapy once a week from which she derived considerable support and encouragement from those members who had been discharged from rehabilitation and were currently experiencing some of the things she anticipated would bar her success at work. Eventually, FC transitioned to a rehabilitation program that was based both at her place of work and at the rehabilitation hospital. In doing so, it was extremely important to modify the attitudinal environment by ensuring that the employer's expectations of FC were commensurate with hers and those of the team. Consequently, the team explained and got the the employer to agree that when FC first returned to work, it would be for the purpose of using the workplace as her rehabilitation medium rather than as functioning as a competitively employed worker. At this stage, rehabilitation shifted from a mode of "hands-on treatment" to one of job coaching, which was carried out by occupational therapy. Within two weeks, the job coaching was discontinued, but FC continued in the group therapy program for a several more months, where she became one who could now encourage others. She was also encouraged by the team at the time of discharge to join the Comebackers Club, a support group for individuals who had suffered a stroke and their families. She remained active in this group for quite some time. While she struggled with her depression for some time after discharge, she did not regress from the outcome of adapted living.

* * * * *

Risk Prevention Plan

Many clients may not present with premorbid or secondary risk conditions or a problematic response to disablement, but instead may hold the potential to develop medical conditions that reduce their quality of life and increase the overall cost of health care if not addressed by the rehabilitation team. Such clients also require a risk prevention plan. The discussion below highlights a few of the most common medical risks that typical rehabilitation clients may be susceptible to and describes preventive measures that health care professionals can follow to control for these factors.

Injuries Resulting from Falls. The average medical bill for emergency treatment of an elderly person's fall is $11,000.[14] There are three main, and preventable, reasons for falls: (1) the disorienting side effects of medications, which often cause a drop in blood pressure that, in turn, results in dizziness, (2) postural hypertension (sharp drop in blood pressure to the brain) that elderly persons can suffer, and (3) a deteriorating sense of balance resulting from erosion in visual and sensory information from the inner ear that is critical for balance.

Clinicians can have a significant impact on reducing the risk of a fall by:

1. identifying clients at risk for falls
2. educating them on the removal of environmental hazards
3. referring to the client's physician to determine whether the client is having an adverse reaction to medications

4. educating clients about the potential adverse affect of their medications on balance if they are not taken properly
5. assisting the client to set up a medication management system
6. educating the client to sit up for a minute or two before getting out of bed
7. educating the client to clench and release the fists and wiggle the ankles throughout the day
8. educating the client regarding safe footwear

Diabetes Mellitus. Diabetes is a common problem in the rehabilitation population. If not properly managed by the client, it can lead to costly secondary complications such as retinopathy, nephropathy, neuropathy, cardiovascular disease, and peripheral vascular disease. Physical exercise is extremely important for those with non–insulin-dependent diabetes.[15] Exercise increases insulin sensitivity, thus improving glucose metabolism, while inactivity decreases insulin resistance. An appropriate exercise program for these clients will improve blood glucose control and reduce cardiovascular risk factors. On the other hand, excessive exercise, especially for those who take insulin, may produce hypoglycemia, cause worsening hyperglycemia, worsen eye complications, produce injuries, and cause cardiac problems. All members of the team can play a significant role in educating their clients regarding these risks.

Stroke. There are a number of controllable stroke risk factors. Diabetes, high blood pressure, atrial fibrillation, high cholesterol, smoking, and alcohol abuse are among them.[16] The risk factors arising from diabetes have been described above. A person with high blood pressure is four to six times more likely to have a stroke. In some cases, blood pressure can be controlled by lifestyle changes, such as losing weight, getting more exercise, reducing sodium intake, or drinking less alcohol. In many instances, atrial fibrillation can be controlled by medication, which requires strict adherence to the prescribed medication regimen. High cholesterol speeds up hardening of the artery walls. Exercising regularly and eating a low-fat diet can help lower cholesterol. Smoking raises blood pressure and increases the likelihood of blood clots. Those who smoke are estimated to be twice as likely to have strokes as nonsmokers; however, several years after quitting smoking, the risk of stroke drops to almost the same level as that of nonsmokers. Heavy alcohol consumption also raises blood pressure, thereby increasing a person's risk of stroke.

Drugs are now available that can significantly reduce the secondary impairments that follow a stroke. To be effective, however, these drugs, which are used for nonhemorrhagic strokes, must be administered within three hours of the onset of symptoms. Thus, it is extremely important to educate clients to seek emergency medical help as soon as they experience early warning signs of stroke such as difficulty talking, or vision difficulties such as sudden blurriness, dimness, an episode of double vision, or loss of vision.

RESOURCE UTILIZATION PLAN

Managing the type, frequency, and duration of therapy is a key component of quality and cost management. In order to manage its resources effectively, the rehabilitation team must establish an individualized resource utilization plan for the client before treatment begins. As the team monitors client progress during the course of rehabilitation, it also monitors and modifies the resource utilization plan to ensure that the most appropriate type of intervention is being provided in the most efficient manner at all times.

Establishing a Resource Utilization Plan

The decision about which resources are needed, when they are needed, and for how long they are needed is based on the following: the client's expected outcome; client/family goals; the client's impairments, functional limitations, and disabilities; as well as the client's ability to benefit from treatment at the moment (i.e., medical, cognitive and/or emotional status, and/or physical or cognitive endurance).

In the process of devising an individualized resource utilization plan for a client, the team needs to answer the following questions:

1. Which disciplines are absolutely required to reduce the client's disabilities?
2. Should all of the client's disabilities be addressed simultaneously, or sequentially?
3. If they are to be addressed sequentially, what is the most appropriate sequence?

4. What frequency, intensity, and duration of treatment should each discipline provide?
5. Should the frequency and intensity of each discipline's treatment be increased or decreased across time; if so, when and how much?
6. Is it appropriate to have services provided by a rehabilitation aide and, if so, when and how much?
7. Can the client benefit from group treatment and/or cotreatment; if so, when and how much?

The individualized resource utilization plan for a given client consists of:

1. the type and level (therapist versus aide) of personnel required to facilitate the attainment of the expected client outcome
2. prioritization of the frequency, amount, and duration of treatment provided by each discipline in relation to the client's current needs and ability to engage in therapy
3. prioritization of the time of day each discipline will treat
4. identification of the service delivery format (e.g., the amount and frequency of individual therapy, cotreatment, rehabilitation technique, and/or group treatment) that will be required to reach the expected outcome and the sequence of their provision

INDIVIDUALIZED CRITICAL PATHWAY

Critical pathways, discussed extensively in Chapter 3, are defined by Coffey as "an optimal sequencing and timing of interventions of health care staff for a particular diagnosis . . . designed to minimize delays and resource utilization, and maximize the quality of care."[17] Critical pathways provide information to the team as to whether a given client's progress is consistent with that of similar clients from the same diagnostic group. This is important quality and cost management information, however, it is not enough. A client's failure to progress in compliance with the generic diagnostic group critical pathway alerts the team to the presence of a problem. However, the client's variation from the pathway does not identify the cause of the problem. Consequently, in addition to the generic critical pathway, the team also needs an individualized critical pathway, a pathway that is based on client-specific skill areas and the degree to which they are expected to have improved by specific points in time across the course of rehabilitation. Discipline-specific short-term goals, when projected for the entire duration of rehabilitation, can be used for this purpose.

Traditionally, therapists do not develop a series of short-term goals that span the entire duration of treatment before treatment begins. Instead, they write short-term goals related to what they expect to occur during a particular brief segment of therapy and then develop the next set of goals at the end of that segment of therapy on the basis of the client's progress. This approach to monitoring progress, however, usually leads to decisions that are made only on the basis of what has occurred during a brief period of time and fail to focus on the total picture. This increases the probability of inappropriate treatment. If one is only looking at a brief time period, it is likely that the therapist will see some degree of progress. The amount and type of progress, however, may not be sufficient to justify continued treatment when measured against the client's initial level of function, the next expected level of function, and the expected outcome. It is entirely possible for a client to make progress from point A to point B during a certain segment of time but not be making progress toward the ultimate outcome. In essence, the therapist becomes more focused on the process of therapy rather than the outcome of that process.

In the MORsystem, each discipline that has been selected to participate in the treatment plan develops short-term goals for the entire expected duration of treatment before it begins. Instead of individual discipline-specific long-terms goals, all short-term goals are related to the client's expected outcome on the Functional Living Scale. Knowing the expected outcome, each discipline forecasts the entire sequence of skills acquisition the client must achieve and the expected time of achievement for each step in the critical pathway that leads to the expected outcome. By forecasting the entire sequence of short-term goals, each discipline has created the blueprint upon which to base the construction of the outcome as well as a method of monitoring progress on the basis of the total picture. As treatment unfolds, short-term goals may be modified when clinically appropriate (e.g., either a positive or negative change in the client's medical or psychological status, the discovery of medical conditions that were previously unknown, a positive or negative change in family support and involvement in the rehabilitation process, and/or a change in the expected place of discharge). Any of these factors can change the expected outcome. When the expected outcome is altered, the short-term goals required to reach it will also be altered. Short-term goals may also be modified because a client's potential abilities initially may have been either over- or underestimated. One must be cautious, however, when employing this reason for modifiying short-term goals. One must be absolutely sure that the goals are not being modified to continue treatment when the client's prognosis does not support such action.

The content of all short-term goals should meet the following criteria:

- It identifies the impairment or functional limitation that will be treated and the expected measurable change that will occur and the length of time it will take to achieve that change.
- It identifies and describes the functional ability that will result from the change that occurs as the impairment or functional limitation decreases.
- It is directly related to the expected outcome.

SHORT-TERM TEAM FOCUS

All clients present with a wide array of impairments, functional limitations, and disabilities. Many clients also present with numerous risk factors. Although all of these factors are barriers to a successful outcome, some are more critical than others. The short-term team focus is that barrier the team has determined to be critical to outcome attainment if not addressed immediately and simultaneously by all team members. Once the team is satisfied that the barrier has been reduced, it identifies the next most critical short-term team focus.

Short-Term Team Focus Examples

- Post–traumatic brain injury client who is a fall risk because of ataxia of gait combined with impulsivity and decreased judgment. *Short-term team focus:* All team members will facilitate the client to scan his environment during activities of daily living and plan his actions before acting, cautiously carry out his plans during activities, and upon task completion immediately review with him the success of the safety measures he has taken.
- Post–brain tumor client who is a fall risk secondary to vertigo. *Short-term team focus:* All team members (a) will facilitate client to identify

his precursors of vertigo, document them in his vertigo tracking log, and identify and document situations/environments that he should avoid and (b) facilitate client to apply the information established in step (a) in the context of his activities of daily living.

- Post–right hemisphere stroke client with hemisensory neglect and at risk to injure the left side of her body as well as general safety risk due to right hemispace neglect. *Short-term team focus:* All team members will cue client to her left side of space by using the phrase "look to your left, now!" while simultaneously providing a tactile cue on her left side and then immediately facilitating her to search for, find, and fixate the red circle attention fixation target. Once target has been attended to, facilitate client to explore the immediate left side environment for safety hazards, verbalize them, and then maneuver around them.

- Post–left hemisphere stroke client who is at risk for right shoulder subluxation. *Short-term team focus:* All team members will facilitate the client to provide proper right arm support and positioning while in the wheelchair, during transfers and ambulation, and when lying down. All team members will also facilitate the daughter's understanding of the importance of proper support and positioning of her father's right arm.

- Post–left hemisphere stroke client whose family is providing more help than he needs. *Short-term team focus:* All team members will decrease family overhelping by providing them both verbally and in writing what the client is able to do for himself without help, what he needs help with, and how much help he will need.

TEAM DISCHARGE PLAN

The team discharge plan describes what must be accomplished by the team, client, and/or family before discharge in order to guarantee that the achieved outcome will be maintained or enhanced after discharge from the client's current level of care. Each identified task is assigned to team members, the client, and family as appropriate and a completion date is set for each task. Progress toward the completion of each task is monitored in all client conferences.

At a minimum, the discharge plan should address the following domains, many of which are included in the Needs-Based Treatment Planning (see Exhibit 4–5):

- Safety
  1. environmental
  2. medical
  3. general health (proper health, recognizing signs of a health problem, carrying out basic first aid)
- Residence
  1. modifications
  2. equipment
  3. supplies
  4. knowledge of alternative residence options and criteria for qualifying
- Family
  1. family/caregiver education and training goals
  2. family/client support systems (e.g., immediate/extended family, friends, their religious and/or organization affiliations)
  3. leisure time resources
  4. respite resources
- Community
  1. vocational
  2. leisure
  3. social
  4. support groups
  5. continued low/no-expense therapy resources
  6. spiritual
  7. transportation
- Financial
  1. resources available within the client's health care policy, how and when to access them, and any restrictions and copayments
  2. local/state/federal resources
  3. how to access these resources

The team discharge plan is not a static document. It is modified during the course of rehabilitation as goals and outcomes are changed. Exhibit 4–7 shows some sample discharge plans.

CONCLUSION

In earlier chapters, it was noted that clinical decisions drive both the quality and cost of rehabilitation. Because of this reality, it is the team that

Exhibit 4–7 Example Discharge Plans

A left hemisphere stroke client who will require considerable caregiver support and the caregiver is at risk for burn-out.

Preliminary discharge plan:
1. Explore the client's and his wife's interest in the adult day healthcare program in their community. If they are interested, facilitate their visit to the program and meeting with the director.
2. Explore the wife's interest in the caregivers' support group provided by our rehabilitation facility. If she is interested, facilitate her attendance at the next meeting.
3. Explore the wife's interest in in-home respite care. If she is interested, facilitate a meeting between her and the director of the Southern Caregivers Association.

A right hemisphere stroke client who is depressed and whose caregiver daughter is at risk for burn-out.

Preliminary discharge plan:
1. Explore the client's interest in the Comebacker's Club (a poststroke peer support group) and facilitate her attendance at the next meeting if she is interested.
2. Explore client's interest in the stress management group provided by this rehabilitation facility and facilitate her attendance at the next meeting if she is interested.
3. Explore the client's interest in returning to her previous involvement in her church. If she is interested, facilitate a meeting between her and her pastor and her occupational therapist to identify previous duties that she may be able to return to at this time.
4. Explore daughter's interest in this rehabilitation facility's caregivers' support group and facilitate her attendance at its next meeting if she so desires.
5. Explore daughter's interest in personal counseling and facilitate an appointment with the social worker if she approves.

A left hemisphere stroke patient who will live alone when discharged and is at risk for depression and physical and communicative regression.

continues

Exhibit 4–7 continued

Preliminary discharge plan:

1. Explore client's interest in volunteer work. If he is interested, facilitate him to identify the type of volunteer work he would prefer, the type of activities within that volunteer work he would be capable of doing, and then facilitate a meeting with the appropriate person at the place of volunteer work.
2. Explore the client's interest in the social activities provided at the senior center in his community. If interested, facilitate a visit to the center and a meeting with its director.
3. Explore the client's interest in the mall walking club that meets at the shopping center near his home. If interested, facilitate a meeting between him and its organizer to learn about its schedule and other activities it undertakes.
4. Assist client to put together a network of family and friends that provide transportation to any of the above-noted activites that he selects.

is in the best position to carry out not only its historical role of quality management, but also to now participate in managing the cost of rehabilitation. To do this, however, the services of all disciplines must be well choreographed, constantly coordinated, continuously monitored, and tightly focused on the same outcome. The traditional approach to service delivery is based on a loose assemblage of noninterlocking discipline-specific goals and treatment plans. This approach will not meet the quality and cost management demands of today. The rehabilitation team is like an orchestra. Each of its members is highly skilled in the techniques of playing different instruments that produce different sounds of great quality. However, in order to produce the music the audience has paid to hear, they all must play from the same score. The client management plan is the rehabilitation team's score. It transcends discipline boundaries and organizes the team around a common goal (outcome) and provides it with the blueprint to guide them in the provision of the right services, in the right amount, at the right time. The success of a client management plan hinges on the viability of the outcome that it is designed to produce. The content of the projected functional living level (i.e., the abilities the client will be able to perform) is determined by the client's disabilities. Once the outcome has been determined, the team is in a position to identify the resources, service delivery format, expected treatment duration, and the level of care that will be needed to reach it. Having codified these quality and cost factors in the form of the client management plan, the team is now in a position to coordinate and continuously monitor its own activities across the course of rehabilitation.

REFERENCES

1. World Health Organization, *International Classification of Impairments, Disabilities, and Handicaps* (Geneva: 1980), 11.
2. National Advisory Board on Medical Rehabilitation and Research, *Draft V: Report and Plan for Medical Rehabilitation Research* (Bethesda, MD: National Institutes of Health, 1992).
3. World Health Organization, *International Classification of Impairments, Disabilities, and Handicaps*, 11.
4. S. Nagi. "Disability Concepts Revisited: Implications for Prevention," in *Disability in America: Toward a National Agenda for Prevention*, eds. A. Pope and A. Tarlov (Washington, DC: National Academy Press, 1991).
5. National Advisory Board on Medical Rehabilitation and Research, *Draft V: Report and Plan for Medical Rehabilitation Research*.
6. O. Payton et al., *Patient Participation in Program Planning: A Manual for Therapists* (Philadelphia: F.A. Davis, 1990).
7. J. Rotter, Generalized Expectancies for Internal versus External Control of Reinforcement, *Psychological Monographs 80*, no. 609 (1966).
8. G. Fawcett et al., Locus of Control, Perceived Constraint, and Moral Among Institutionalized Aged, *International Journal Aging and Human Development 11*, no. 1 (1980).
9. M. Seligman, *Helplessness: On Depression, Development, and Death* (San Francisco: W.H. Freeman & Co., 1975).
10. Nagi, "Disability Concepts Revisited."
11. M. Brown et al., "Rehabilitation Indicators," in *Functional Assessment in Rehabilitation*, ed. A.S. Fuhrer (Baltimore: Paul H. Brookes Publishing, 1984), 187–203.
12. A.M. Pope and A.R. Tarlov, eds., *Disability in America: Toward a National Agenda for Prevention* (Washington, DC: National Academy Press, 1991), 8.
13. L. Verbrugge and A. Jette, *The Disablement Process, Society of Science and Medicine 38* (1994): 1–14.
14. S. Allis et al., *Aging 85*, no. 12 (1996), 78–80.
15. D. Slovik, Diabetes and Rehab, *Rehab Management* February/March (1997): 46.
16. R. Dinsmoor, Stroke, What It Is and What To Do, *Diabetes Self-Management* September/October (1996): 60.
17. R. Coffey et al., An Introduction to Critical Paths, *Quality Management in Health Care 1*, no. 1 (1992): 45–54.

Appendix 4–A
Client/Family Request for Services

INSTRUCTIONS: Tell us which abilities you would like to improve by putting a circle around either yes or no next to each ability.

Tell us how important it is to you to have this ability improved by putting a check (✓) in the box next to either:

Important		☐
Very Important		☐
Extremely Important		☐

Activities Done in the Home

	ABILITY		IMPORTANCE	
1	Improve his/her ability to move in/out/around the bed?	Yes/No	Important	☐
			Very Important	☐
			Extremely Important	☐
2	Improve his/her ability to sit/stand/walk/move from one position to another?	Yes/No	Important	☐
			Very Important	☐
			Extremely Important	☐
3	Improve his/her ability to manage the wheelchair or other adaptive equipment.	Yes/No	Important	☐
			Very Important	☐
			Extremely Important	☐
4	Improve his/her ability to dress/bathe/groom/feed/medicate himself/herself or with using the toilet?	Yes/No	Important	☐
			Very Important	☐
			Extremely Important	☐
5	Decrease the amount of time he/she spends not doing anything?	Yes/No	Important	☐
			Very Important	☐
			Extremely Important	☐
6	Change the amount of time he/she watches television, listen to the radio, looks outside?	Yes/No	Important	☐
			Very Important	☐
			Extremely Important	☐
7	Increase the amount of time he/she exercises?	Yes/No	Important	☐
			Very Important	☐
			Extremely Important	☐
8	Improve his/her ability to do activities such as reading books, playing solitaire, working puzzles, doing handwork, playing a musical instrument, working with a computer, playing video games?	Yes/No	Important	☐
			Very Important	☐
			Extremely Important	☐
9	Improve his/her ability to do household chores, cooking or gardening?	Yes/No	Important	☐
			Very Important	☐
			Extremely Important	☐

Activities Done in the Home

	ABILITY		IMPORTANCE	
10	Improve his/her ability to care for children/grandchildren?	Yes/No	Important Very Important Extremely Important	❏ ❏ ❏
11	Improve his/her ability to know what to do in an emergency?	Yes/No	Important Very Important Extremely Important	❏ ❏ ❏
12	Are there any other routine/daily activities that you would like assistance with? If yes, write the activity here:	Yes/No	Important Very Important Extremely Important	❏ ❏ ❏

Activities Done Outside the Home

	ABILITY		IMPORTANCE	
1	Improve his/her ability to use public transportation?	Yes/No	Important Very Important Extremely Important	❏ ❏ ❏
2	Improve his/her ability to drive a car?	Yes/No	Important Very Important Extremely Important	❏ ❏ ❏
3	Improve his/her ability to keep appointments (such as with doctor/dentist/programs)?	Yes/No	Important Very Important Extremely Important	❏ ❏ ❏
4	Improve his/her ability to take walks/go to the park/shopping mall/beach?	Yes/No	Important Very Important Extremely Important	❏ ❏ ❏
5	Improve his/her ability to attend religious/club services or events?	Yes/No	Important Very Important Extremely Important	❏ ❏ ❏
6	Improve his/her ability to go to a movie, other cultural or sporting events?	Yes/No	Important Very Important Extremely Important	❏ ❏ ❏
7	Improve his/her ability to go to a restaurant and with ordering/paying for meals?	Yes/No	Important Very Important Extremely Important	❏ ❏ ❏
8	Improve his/her ability to shop or run errands?	Yes/No	Important Very Important Extremely Important	❏ ❏ ❏

	ABILITY		IMPORTANCE	
9	Improve his/her ability to budget and manage his/her money?	Yes/No	Important Very Important Extremely Important	☐ ☐ ☐
10	Improve his/her ability to read/write, attend school, use the library?	Yes/No	Important Very Important Extremely Important	☐ ☐ ☐
11	Are there other activities done outside the living situation that you would like assistance with? If yes, write the activity here:	Yes/No	Important Very Important Extremely Important	☐ ☐ ☐

Regular Community Activities

	ABILITY		IMPORTANCE	
1	Would you like assistance with going to a support group?	Yes/No	Important Very Important Extremely Important	☐ ☐ ☐
2	Improve his/her ability to go to parks and recreation program / center?	Yes/No	Important Very Important Extremely Important	☐ ☐ ☐
3	Improve his/her ability to do volunteer work in the community? If yes, what kind of work?	Yes/No	Important Very Important Extremely Important	☐ ☐ ☐
4	Improve his/her ability to obtain gainful employment. If yes, what kind of work?	Yes/No	Important Very Important Extremely Important	☐ ☐ ☐
5	Are there any other activities done regularly outside the living situation that you would like assistance with? If yes, write the activity here:	Yes/No	Important Very Important Extremely Important	☐ ☐ ☐

Activities Done to Maintain Relationships With Others

	ABILITY		IMPORTANCE	
1	Improve his/her ability to talk on the telephone, find numbers in the phone book, dial numbers?	Yes/No	Important Very Important Extremely Important	☐ ☐ ☐

	ABILITY		IMPORTANCE	
2	Improve his/her ability to write letters, or select and send cards?	Yes/No	Important Very Important Extremely Important	☐ ☐ ☐
3	Improve his/her ability to talk with members of the family?	Yes/No	Important Very Important Extremely Important	☐ ☐ ☐
4	Improve his/her ability to talk with friends?	Yes/No	Important Very Important Extremely Important	☐ ☐ ☐
5	Increase his/her ability to talk with new people?	Yes/No	Important Very Important Extremely Important	☐ ☐ ☐
6	Would you like assistance with his/her sexual activity?	Yes/No	Important Very Important Extremely Important	☐ ☐ ☐
7	Improve ability to control his/her feelings?	Yes/No	Important Very Important Extremely Important	☐ ☐ ☐
8	Are there any other activities which assist in developing/maintaining social contrats that you would like assistance with? If yes, write the activity here:	Yes/No	Important Very Important Extremely Important	☐ ☐ ☐

‾‾‾‾‾‾‾‾‾‾‾‾‾‾‾‾‾‾‾   ‾‾‾‾‾‾‾‾‾‾‾‾‾‾‾‾‾‾‾
Program Representative   Family Member

‾‾‾‾‾‾‾‾‾‾‾‾‾‾‾‾‾‾‾   ‾‾‾‾‾‾‾‾‾‾‾‾‾‾‾‾‾‾‾
Date   Relationship

CHAPTER 5

Process Management Tools

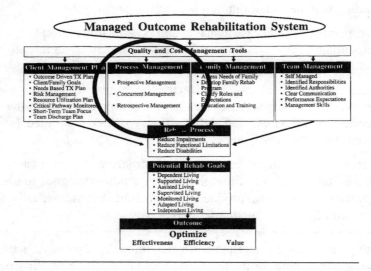

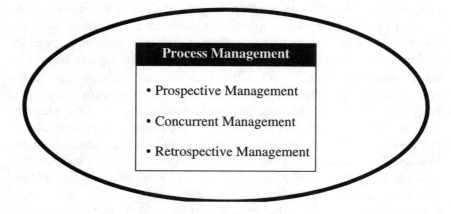

Process Management

- Prospective Management

- Concurrent Management

- Retrospective Management

KEY POINTS

- Quality and cost management are based on the consistent provision of good rehabilitation services, the avoidance of futile rehabilitation services, and the elimination of bad rehabilitation services.

- Prospective clinical case management avoids futile care by determining whether rehabilitation is medically necessary.

- Prospective clinical case management lays the foundation for good rehabilitation services through the establishment of an interdisciplinary client treatment plan.

- Concurrent clinical case management ensures the provision of good rehabilitation services through the continuous monitoring of service effectiveness and determining whether continued rehabilitation is medically necessary.

- Retrospective clinical case management strives to eliminate bad rehabilitation services through outcome studies designed to identify those services that produce the best clinical, customer satisfaction, and financial outcomes.

Quality and cost management are not mutually exclusive activities. Producing an outcome for the least cost does not mean that quality of care must be sacrificed. On the contrary, good quality management systems and procedures will result in good cost management. Quality services are those services that produce an outcome that is meaningful and utilitarian in the client's natural environment, that is retained over time without the need for further intervention, and reduces the risk for future complications. To achieve these outcomes, the rehabilitation team must clinically manage the type, frequency, and duration of treatment; the service delivery format (e.g., individual, dual, group, and aide-provided services); and the client's level of care, as well as risk for complications. The rehabilitation team will achieve the best outcome from a quality perspective when it matches the above management activities with the client's existing needs and ability to participate meaningfully in and gain advantage from rehabilitation intervention. The team concurrently must address those risks that either are current barriers to improvement or that represent future problems that could result in the loss of gains made through rehabilitation after discharge.

All of these clinical decisions are both quality and cost management decisions. From a clinical decision-making perspective, the team has three quality and cost management responsibilities. They must ensure: (1) the consistent provision of good care, (2) the avoidance of futile care, and (3) the elimination of bad care.

The consistent provision of good care is fundamental to producing an outcome with a good cost/benefit ratio. It is equally apparent that the provision of services to those who cannot benefit from them and the provision of inappropriate or ineffective services will result in an outcome with a poor cost/benefit ratio. The fundamental issue, then, in quality and cost management is to ensure that services are provided by the appropriate personnel, to the appropriate people, at the appropriate level of care, at the appropriate time, for the appropriate length of time.

The Managed Outcome Rehabilitation System (MORsystem) is based on the premise that, to produce the best outcome for the least cost, the rehabilitation team can and must objectively manage the course of rehabilitation both prospectively (i.e., before treatment begins) and concurrently (while treatment is being provided) as well as improve the future process of providing rehabilitation services retrospectively through outcome studies.

Prospective case management involves:

- providing rehabilitation services only to clients who have been identified as holding the potential to benefit from such services, and
- organizing the team's activities around a non–discipline-specific client management plan that is tightly focused on what will be required either to discharge the client from rehabilitation or to transfer the client to the next least intense level of care as quickly as possible

Concurrent case management involves:

- focusing treatment on those disabilities that must be reduced in order to transfer the client to the next level of care or to meet the client's needs in his or her "real world" discharge environment,
- focusing treatment on those impairments or functional limitations that are directly related to the target disabilities,
- matching the frequency and intensity of each discipline's interventions in relation to the client's prevailing needs,

- prioritizing the frequency and intensity of each discipline's interventions in relation to the client's cognitive, emotional, and/or physical ability to gain a therapeutic advantage from intervention at any given point in time, and
- continually monitoring the medical necessity of treatment.

Retrospective case management involves:

- the evaluation of the success of rehabilitation in relation to previously established quality outcome indicators
- the identification of the "best practices" (i.e., those practices that have a strong correlation with successful outcomes)
- the identification of "futile practices" (i.e., those practices that did not make a difference in the outcome)
- the identification of "bad practices" (i.e., those practices that have a strong correlation with unsuccessful outcomes)
- the dissemination of information regarding good, futile, and bad practices to facilitate continuous improvement of the quality of rehabilitation

PROSPECTIVE CASE MANAGEMENT

Prospective quality and cost management is the process of determining whether rehabilitation is "medically necessary" and, if it is, to decide whether the client is at the level of care appropriate to meet his or her rehabilitation needs. The purpose of determining medical necessity is to ensure that the team does not provide unnecessary or futile care. While clients are typically screened for rehabilitation potential prior to admission to rehabilitation, the fact that the client has been admitted should not be taken as prima facie evidence that rehabilitation is in fact medically necessary.

To determine whether rehabilitation is medically necessary, the team evaluates its assessment findings in relationship to the following questions:

1. Has the client had a medical episode that has resulted in impairments, functional limitations, and disabilities?

2. Have the impairments, functional limitations, and disabilities significantly decreased the client's level of function compared with his or her level of function prior to the medical episode?
3. Is rehabilitation reasonable and necessary in relation to the client's condition? That is, does the client's impairments and functional limitations cause a disability, a gap, between the client's performance abilities and those that are required to function in his or her living environment? If they do not, then rehabilitation is neither reasonable nor necessary. Conversely, if the client's impairments and functional limitations have resulted in a disability, will rehabilitation yield significant practical improvement? That is, is the severity of the client's impairments and functional limitations of such a magnitude that rehabilitation will result in an increase in performance abilities sufficient to meet the demands of the client's natural living environment?

Once the team has determined that rehabilitation is medically necessary, it must then determine whether the client is at the appropriate level of care. Just as admission to rehabilitation does not automatically mean that it is medically necessary, neither should it be assumed that the admission level of care best meets the client's needs.

In addition to using the level of care criteria presented in Chapter 3, the team must also determine the appropriate level of care on the basis of the following questions:

- Are the type of services that can be provided at this level of care specific to the client's condition?
- Will the amount and frequency of services provided at this level of care be appropriate for the client's condition?

Client Management Plan

It cannot be stated often enough that a map without a destination or a destination without a map are both useless. To manage the course of rehabilitation, members of the team must know where they are going collectively before rehabilitation begins and they must have an objective guidance mechanism that will tell them whether they are making progress toward their destination and whether they will reach it on time. Prospective clinical case management is the process of establishing what the team expects to achieve (the destination) for a given client as well as identifying objective clinical criteria (a map) by which to monitor the client's progress toward that outcome before (prospectively) rehabilitation begins. The client management plan (CMP) embodies the team's destination and the map they will use to guide themselves to that destination in an effective and timely manner. The CMP is the team's prospective clinical management tool. Developed before treatment begins, it is the blueprint that specifies what the outcome should be, and what skills and functional abilities must be acquired, and when they are expected to be acquired in order to meet the expected outcome.

The CMP is developed in the first client conference and modified in follow-up conferences as clinically indicated. It involves an 11-step process, which is outlined here and described in more detail below. The CMP consists of:

- the client's prior level of function
- the client's current level of function
- expected outcome
- risk factors
- client/family goals
- specific disabilities, functional limitations, and impairments that must be reduced to support the expected outcome
- short-term goals for each discipline
- an individualized resource utilization plan
- short-term team focus
- family and education training goals
- preliminary discharge plan

Step 1: Identify the Client's Prior Level of Function

The team selects from the Functional Living Scale (see Exhibit 4–4) the level of function that best describes the client's ability to perform his or her usual and customary daily living skills prior to the medical episode.

Step 2: Identify the Client's Current Level of Function

The team establishes the client's current level of function by selecting the level of function from the Functional Living Scale (see Exhibit 4–4) that best describes the client's level of function at the time of the team's initial evaluations.

Step 3: Identify the Client's Expected Outcome

The team selects the projected outcome from the Functional Living Scale (see Exhibit 4–4) based on the following parameters:

- length, type, and frequency of treatment authorized by the client's health care benefits plan
- type and level of daily living skills the client wants to be able to perform
- type and level of daily living skills the family will allow the client to perform
- degree of family support
- expected degree to which the client's impairments/functional limitations can be reduced

Step 4: Identify Risk Factors

The team identifies any premorbid or secondary conditions, response to disablement, and/or environmental factors that could be potential barriers to the attainment of the projected outcome or could potentially cause regression from that outcome after discharge.

Step 5: Establish Client/Family Goals

Given the expected outcome, the team determines the specific abilities that the client and family want the client to be able to perform.

Step 6: Identify Impairments and Disabilities

The team determines which impairments are causing any disabilities. Of those identified impairments, the team next decides which will require the knowledge, skills, and judgment of a therapist in order to improve and which hold the greatest potential to improve.

Based on client and family goals and assessment results, the team selects from the Individualized Daily Living Skills checklist (see Exhibit 4–6) those daily living skills that the client will be required to master in order to compensate for any disabilities and in order to function in the client's place of residence.

Step 7: Develop Short-Term Goals for Each Discipline

Each discipline develops short-term goals for each of the disabilities that has been selected. Short-term goals are developed for the entire length of stay. Each discipline writes its short-term goals for the initial conference and provides them to the case manager at the time of the conference.

Step 8: Identify Individualized Resource Utilization Plan

The team next determines the type and level (therapist versus aide) of personnel that will be required to facilitate the client's attainment of the expected outcome. The team prioritizes the frequency, amount, and duration of treatment that will be provided by each discipline in relation to the client's current needs and ability to engage in therapy. It then identifies the service delivery format (e.g., the amount and frequency of individual, dual, or group treatment) that will be required to reach the expected outcome and the sequence of service provision.

Step 9: Establish Short-Term Team Focus

Most clients will present with a multitude of clinical problems (e.g., risk factors, impairments, functional limitations, and disabilities) that must be successfully addressed in order to attain the expected outcome. However, one or two of these problems will be more immediate, critical barriers to outcome acquisition than the others. The team identifies these critical barriers, and each member of the team focuses on them within the context of his or her discipline-specific treatment session. The team identifies its short-term team focus by posing the following question: Of all of the client's problems, which one or two are the greatest barriers to progress at this time, and which barriers, if focused on by all disciplines for a brief period of time, will accelerate progress toward the expected outcome?

Step 10: Develop Family Education and Training Goals

Each discipline develops time-framed and measurable short-term goals that focus on what the caregiver will need to know and be able to do in order to support the client's achieved abilities after discharge.

Step 11: Prepare Preliminary Discharge Plan

This plan identifies what must be accomplished by the team, client, and/ or family before discharge in order to ensure that the achieved outcome is maintained or enhanced after discharge. At minimum, the discharge plan should address individualized needs in the following domains: health safety, residence, family, community, and financial.

The development of the CMP should take no longer than 30 minutes. To accomplish this, each member of the team must have completed the following tasks prior to the initial conference:

1. determined what they believe the client's current level of function and expected outcome level of function to be
2. identified the client's functional limitations, impairments, and disabilities
3. determined preliminary client/family education and training needs
4. identified preliminary discharge needs

Having prepared in advance, each therapist should readily be able to focus on, discuss, and reach consensus on each of these elements of the CMP. The case manager identifies client/family goals prior to the conference and presents them at the conference. The client's service delivery format and short-term team focus are established at the time of the conference, based on the team's discussion of the expected outcome, client/family goals, and the client's functional limitations, impairments, and disabilities.

Quality and cost management requires the team's movement away from the traditional multidisciplinary service model to a highly integrated approach to service delivery—an interdisciplinary team approach. The processes involved in the development and implementation of the CMP

facilitates a team's evolution from a multidisciplinary to an interdisciplinary approach to service delivery. In the multidisciplinary team approach
(Figure 5–1), each discipline independently establishes its specific long-
and short-term goals, patient/family education and training goals, and
discharge plan. Inherently, the multidisciplinary service delivery model
"segments" the client and creates gaps in service delivery as well as the
potential for duplication of services. This approach also holds the potential
for slow progress during rehabilitation and client regression from the
discipline outcomes after discharge. It presumes that the client and the
client's family will somehow understand the relationships among the goals
of each discipline and figure out how everything fits together to produce
integrated functional daily living skills by or after discharge. An interdis-

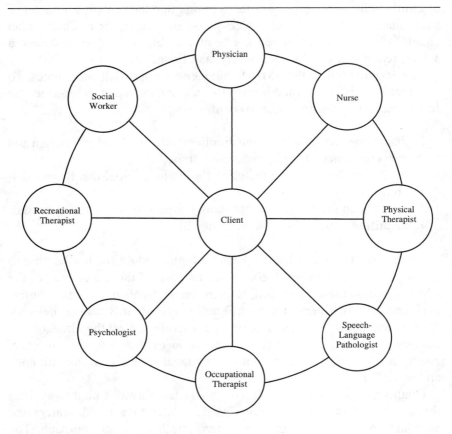

Figure 5–1 Multidisciplinary Team Approach

ciplinary team approach (Figure 5–2) organizes and manages all discipline interventions around a common outcome, treatment plan, client/family education and training plan, and discharge plan. Each discipline's short-term goals are focused on, linked to and directed toward these four common components of the treatment plan.

In the MORsystem, the expected outcome is the long-term goal for all disciplines. By establishing a single non–discipline-specific outcome (i.e., long-term goal), all team members focus their respective discipline-specific treatments on a common effort. This increases the continuity of treatment across all disciplines as well as the client's understanding of the linkage among the various therapies, goals, and treatment approaches.

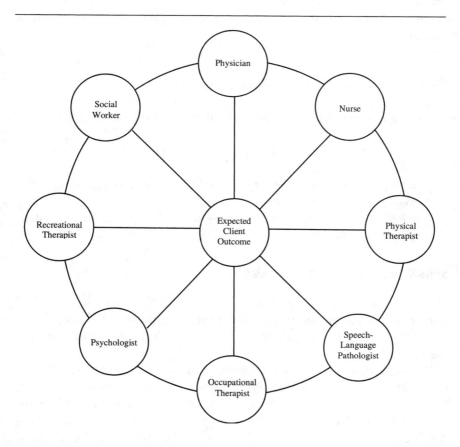

Figure 5–2 Interdisciplinary Team Approach

When continuity and client understanding are increased, the power of the rehabilitation effort is also significantly intensified.

CONCURRENT CLINICAL CASE MANAGEMENT

Concurrent clinical case management is the process of continually monitoring a client's progress once rehabilitation has commenced for the purpose of determining whether continued rehabilitation is medically necessary. Continued treatment is based on the determination that treatment continues to be reasonable and necessary to the client's condition. Treatment is reasonable and necessary when it is consistent with the diagnosis and when its omission would adversely affect the client's condition or quality of life.

Medical Necessity Decision-Making Process

The team uses three criteria to determine medical necessity:

1. whether the client is making significant practical improvement toward the expected outcome
2. whether skilled services are required to sustain progress toward the expected outcome
3. whether the client's current level of care is required to sustain progress toward the expected outcome

Significant Practical Improvement

A substantial and measurable decrease in the client's current level of impairment or functional limitation compared to his or her admission level of impairment or functional limitation constitutes a significant improvement.

Practical improvement is defined as a substantial and measurable increase in the client's ability to perform—outside the direction and support of a clinician and/or therapeutic environment—those safety, health maintenance, personal care, household management, community access, productive activity, and/or leisure skills the team, client, and family have identified as necessary for the client to function within the client's living environment.

Continued rehabilitation is reasonable and necessary to the client's condition as long as there is objective evidence that therapy services are either reducing impairments with a concomitant significant reduction in the client's functional limitations, or are reducing functional limitations with a concomitant significant in reduction of the client's disabilities. The reduction of impairments without a reduction of functional limitations or a reduction in functional limitations without an increase in the client's ability to perform targeted daily living skills indicates that continued rehabilitation is not reasonable and necessary to the client's condition.

Continued treatment is justified (medically necessary) if the client's current level of function represents a significant practical improvement from his or her admission level of function and the current level of function represents a significant improvement toward the expected outcome level of function.

Objective Evidence of Significant Practical Improvement

The determination of significant practical improvement is not based solely on progress toward discipline-specific short-term goals. It is made on the basis of evidence that indicates that improvement at the micro level of change (discipline short-term goals) is, in fact, resulting in concurrent positive change at the macro, or "whole person" level. For it is progress toward the whole person (i.e., the client's expected outcome) level of function that is the true measure of significant practical improvement. As depicted in Exhibit 5–1, it is expected, depending upon type and severity of impairments, that the client will progress across one, two, or all three phases of rehabilitation to achieve his or her expected outcome. Depending upon the expected outcome, each discipline establishes impairment reduction, functional limitation reduction, and disability reduction short-term goals before treatment begins. These short-term goals focus only on those daily living skills that the client must be able to perform in order to meet the demands of his or her natural environment. The team monitors and measures the rate and degree of progress across the three following macro level indicators of significant practical improvement to ensure that progress, as measured by discipline-specific short-term goals, is resulting in continuous practical improvement toward the expected outcome: (1) the

Exhibit 5–1 Concurrent Clinical Case Management

Phases of Rehab	Impairment Reduction →		Functional Limitation Reduction →		Disability Reduction →			Expected Outcomes
Phases of Intervention	Hands-On Treatment		Coach & Guide		Monitor & Feedback			
Phases of Learning	Unable to purposefully participate in rehabilitation or remember therapy goals and instructions	Understands therapy goals and process but requires continuous repetition of instructions and cueing to initiate and complete rehab tasks	Self-initiated participation in therapy with intermittent ability to self-direct sustained efforts toward therapy goals	Self-initiated and sustained efforts toward therapy goals in structured treatment environment	Carry over newly learned abilities in nontreatment environment with minimum assistance	Generalization of learned abilities to new/unexpected tasks with standby assistance	Carry over newly learned tasks & generalization independently	Independent Living / Adapted Living / Monitored Living
Phases of Functional Change	Performs less than 25% of personal care and leisure living skills	Performs at least 25% of personal care, community access, and leisure living skills	Performs 50%–75% of personal care, household management, community access and leisure living skills	Performs 75% or more of daily living skills	Performs all daily living skills with occasional assistance	Independent in all daily living skills but requires an assistive device, environmental modifications, compensatory strategies, and/or more than usual amount of time to perform daily living activities	Independent in all daily living skills	Supervised Living / Assisted Living / Supported Living
Required Daily Living Skills			Expected Phases of Individualized Skills Recovery					
Safety	STG*	STG	STG	STG	STG	STG		Dependent Living
Health Mainten.	STG	STG	STG	STG	STG	STG		
Personal Care	STG	STG	STG	STG	STG	STG		
Household Management	STG	STG	STG	STG	STG	STG		
Community Access	STG	STG	STG	STG	STG	STG		
Productivity Activity	STG	STG	STG	STG	STG	STG		
Leisure Activity	STG	STG	STG	STG	STG	STG		
Staffing	Modified across time relative to client needs							Total Care

*Short-term goals

phases of treatment intervention, (2) the phases of learning, and (3) phases of functional change. If improvement at the level of short-term goals is facilitating significant practical improvement at the whole person level, one would expect to see the client's ever increasing ability to understand the purpose of his or her goals, ability to self-initiate and sustain effort toward them (i.e., decreasing dependence on cues and structure provided by the therapist) and generalization of abilities learned in relation to specific treatment tasks to similar tasks that occur outside of treatment sessions. One would also expect progress across the phases of learning to be concurrently reflected in commensurate progress across the phases of functional change. Finally, one would expect to see an ever decreasing frequency and amount of therapy provided to a client as he or she progresses across the three phases of treatment intervention. Each phase of treatment intervention requires a different type and amount of intervention. Impairment reduction, the facilitation and stabilization of isolated skill, requires intensive direct hands-on treatment. For example, achieving independent dynamic standing balance, increasing right hand grip strength, or increasing an apraxic's ability to produce isolated words all require hands-on intervention. Functional limitation reduction, the integration of isolated skills into functional abilities, requires less intensive hands-on treatment and more frequent coaching and guiding. For example, challenging the client's dynamic standing balance within the context of transfers, or grip strength within the context of grasping and holding eating utensils, or producing a three-word phrase to describe a picture depicting a common activity of daily living, and providing the ongoing cues and periodic hands-on facilitation necessary for the client to successfully perform these tasks. Disability reduction, facilitating the client to apply regained functional skills in the context of meeting real-life needs, is the least intense phase of treatment intervention. For example, monitoring and providing feedback to the client regarding dynamic standing balance while grocery shopping, or gripping and holding eating utensils while eating in the cafeteria, or explaining his or her health concerns during a visit with the doctor. Not only do clients require less frequent intervention during the disability reduction phase of rehabilitation, they also do not require the involvement of the same number of disciplines as before. By the time the client has reached this phase of rehabilitation, one or two disciplines can provide the required monitoring and feedback related to all of the disciplines' treatment focus and goals.

Thus, as depicted in Exhibit 5–1, significant practical improvement is determined by applying a clinical case management "means test" to the discipline-specific short-term goals and to the phases of functional change, learning, treatment intervention, and rehabilitation. That is, at any given point in time, the team measures whether the client's level of function, as reflected in these five indexes of improvement, matches the level of performance the team predicted would occur at that point in time. The team uses their responses to the following seven questions to measure a client's actual level of performance in relation to the expected level of performance:

1. Is the client's performance on treatment tasks the same or greater than the performance expectations stated in the short-term goals?
2. Is the client achieving the short-term goals at or before the expected time of achievement?
3. Is the client's phase of learning commensurate with the progress reflected in the short-term goals?
4. Is the client's phase of functional change commensurate with the progress reflected in both the phase of learning and the short-term goals?
5. Is the client progressing through the expected phases of rehabilitation?
6. Is the client progressing through the expected phases of treatment?
7. Is the frequency and intensity of staff utilization decreasing across the three phases of rehabilitation and treatment?

If the answer to all of these questions is "yes," then the client is making significant practical improvement and continued rehabilitation is medically necessary to the client's condition. This clinical decision-making matrix indicates that progress in achieving short-term goals (specific progress indicators) alone is not a sufficient determinant of the medical necessity of continued rehabilitation. Medical necessity must also be based on a demonstrated concurrent and measurable linkage between the isolated specific progress indicators and the general progress indicators and, that the type and degree of progress across the continuum of both specific and general progress indicators is leading to what the client will require in order to function at the expected outcome level of living.

For example, if a client is achieving the established short-term goals but is not demonstrating the level of learning and performance that one would expect to result from that improvement, it may indicate that the client is at a maintenance level of care—that is, the client is able to perform higher level skills only within the context of the structure, cues, and motivation of a therapy environment. As such, therapy is creating and maintaining a level of function that the client cannot replicate outside of that environment. In another example, a client may be demonstrating progress in short-term goal acquisition and a commensurate increase in learning and functional change during the impairment reduction phase of rehabilitation, but is not able to do so when the therapists decrease the frequency and intensity of hands-on treatment and move to the coach and guide treatment phase. Again, this may indicate that the client has reached a maintenance level of care and, therefore, rehabilitation is no longer medically necessary. It is also possible that a client is making significant practical improvement in both specific and general progress indicators but that degree of progress is not leading toward abilities that will be required for the client to function at the expected outcome level of living. Finally, the number of staff involved in a client's rehabilitation and the frequency and intensity of their treatment should decrease as the client moves across the phases of rehabilitation, treatment, learning, and functional change. A client may not be making significant practical improvement if these staffing variables remain the same.

A "no" response to any of the seven questions posed above does not mean that the client is automatically discharged from rehabilitation. Instead, the failure to pass one of these clinical means tests is first and foremost a signal that the team must immediately determine the reasons for the client's lack of significant practical improvement. To do this, each clinician and the team as a whole evaluate the client's status at the follow-up client conference in relation to the following questions:

- What interventions and outcomes should be happening at this time?
- What is actually happening?
- What didn't happen and why?
- What should be done?
    1. Should the rehabilitation program continue as planned?
    2. Should the frequency, amount, or duration of treatment provided by one or more disciplines be increased/decreased?
    3. Should the treatment provided by one or more disciplines be discontinued?
    4. Should the resource utilization plan be modified?

5. Should the expected outcome be modified downward?
6. Should the client be discharged to another level of care?
7. Should the client be discharged from rehabilitation?

A client should be discharged from rehabilitation if the team determines that the answer to all of these questions, except the last one, is "no." A "no" response to these questions means that the team has evaluated the treatment program and determined that it is appropriate and, therefore, the lack of significant practical improvement does not lie in the area of service provision but rather with the client's inability to benefit from it. On the other hand, the treatment plan should be redesigned and treatment should continue if it is determined that the treatment program, as originally designed, is not appropriate to the client's needs as they are now understood. If the expected outcome is lowered, it would be expected that the duration of the program would also be less and, consequently, there would be significant changes in the individualized resource utilization plan.

Skilled Services Required To Sustain Progress

A second determinant of medical necessity is whether skilled services are required to sustain progress toward the expected client outcome. There is neither a single nor an arbitrary distinction between skilled and nonskilled services. Instead, this decision must be based on both *static* and *dynamic* definitions of skilled services. The *static* definition describes *what* constitutes skilled services (e.g., the required knowledge and skills). The *dynamic* definition describes *when* such services are skilled (e.g., rendering professional judgment about whether a patient is making significant, practical improvement).

Static Definition of Skilled Services

A static definition of skilled services includes those services that:

- are based on a formal course of academic and clinical preparation
- are related to a medical condition
- are directed toward the amelioration of impairments and/or disabilities for the purpose of reducing safety risks, preventing secondary complications, and/or facilitating a client's attainment of daily living independence that is higher than his or her existing level of independence

- Require a therapist's knowledge and skills to:
  1. evaluate, identify, and measure the impairments, functional limitations, and disabilities caused by the medical condition
  2. establish measurable functional outcome goals
  3. establish a treatment plan that is designed to facilitate the client's attainment of the outcome goals
  4. establish a client/family education and training plan
  5. implement the treatment plan and the client/family education plan
  6. monitor client progress toward the outcome goals and adjust the treatment plan when indicated in order to ensure the client's attainment of the outcome goals
  7. determine when a client has either met the established goals, or no longer requires skilled services to continue progress toward the outcome goals, or can no longer benefit from any level of service
  8. develop and implement a maintenance program and, if needed, periodically reevaluate the client to determine whether the program needs to be modified, and to make appropriate modifications when indicated

Dynamic Definition of Skilled Services

The services described above are considered to be skilled when, in the judgment of the therapist:

- the client holds a prognosis to attain a level of function that is significantly higher than his or her existing level and that the client will be able to maintain that level of function in the absence of continued therapeutic intervention
- the services will and do reduce disabilities
- the services will and do produce continuous significant practical improvement in a client's level of functional independence
- the services will and do result in a client's movement from a more intense level of care to a less intense level of care

Nonskilled Services

A client may meet the static definition for the need for skilled services but not the dynamic criteria that indicate that skilled services are reasonable and necessary to the client's condition. This usually occurs when one of the following conditions occur:

- The client holds the potential to continue to progress but continued progress is not dependent upon continued skilled services. In such instances, the therapist determines that the client's continuation of the home exercise program under the supervision of a family member and the therapeutic benefits that accrue from participation in daily living activities will adequately support the continuation of progress.

- All therapy goals have been met and it is determined that the client does not hold the potential to benefit from treatment toward new goals but does require assistance from another to maintain the level of function that has been achieved.

- It is determined that the client is not making significant practical improvement toward the expected outcome but does require assistance from another to maintain the level of function that has been achieved.

Continued therapist intervention when any of these conditions exist would be considered inappropriate since the client now needs nonskilled maintenance care. It is the responsibility of the therapists to apply both the static and dynamic criteria of skilled care and use their clinical judgment to identify the point at which skilled care is no longer reasonable and necessary to the client's condition. In this regard, it is important to recognize the clinical reality that some clients with medical conditions resulting in impairments and disabilities either will not require or will not benefit from skilled intervention. Some clients may improve without intervention and others will not benefit from rehabilitation, regardless of the type and amount provided. Further, of those who require skilled intervention, not all require it throughout the entire course of their rehabilitation. Finally, the mere provision of a skilled service, in accordance with its static definition, does not in and of itself mean that the service is skilled. Depending upon a client's response to therapy, the intervention required may be skilled services at one point in time and nonskilled at another. The bottom line is that the therapist must exercise expert clinical judgment based on objective clinical findings.

Level of Care

The third medical necessity criterion is whether the client is receiving services at the appropriate level of care. Once it has been determined that the client is making significant practical improvement and that skilled services are required to continue such progress toward the expected outcome, the team must then ask a third question: Is this the appropriate level of care? That is, is the rehabilitation intensity provided at the present level of care absolutely necessary to sustain continued significant practical improvement? As described in Chapter 4, the team bases its decision not only on the knowledge of the admission and discharge criteria for the client's present level of care, but also the knowledge of the admission and discharge criteria for all other levels of care. With this knowledge, the team can compare its clinical knowledge of the client's current and expected future needs and abilities and select from the menu of levels of care that one that will sustain progress with the least intense utilization of resources.

RETROSPECTIVE CASE MANAGEMENT

The purpose of prospective and concurrent clinical case management is to ensure that the clients who are receiving rehabilitation today are receiving the most effective and efficient services possible—that the right staff are providing the right service, to the right person, in the right amount, for the right length of time, at the right time, and at the right level of care. The purpose of retrospective clinical case management is to ensure that those who will require rehabilitation in the future receive services that are more effective and efficient than those provided today. Because knowledge, technology, and the demands for greater effectiveness and efficiency will continue to increase, achieving a higher degree of quality of care cannot be conceived of as a static goal that remains constant once achieved. Achieving the highest quality of care is the therapist's ongoing goal that will never be completely met; yet the act of seeking it will continually improve the services rendered.

The quality of care question posed in the past was: "Does what we do produce results?" The question asked today is quite different: "Do the results we produce make a difference?" Those who pay for health care services and those who receive them want to know: "What is the value, the worth, of rehabilitation services?" All of these stakeholders ensure quality; they seek value. That which constitutes a desirable outcome must be based on a value system, a system that includes all stakeholders.

Defining Quality and Value: Three Perspectives

The continual quest to provide the highest quality of service is not foreign to rehabilitation professionals; the concept of value, however, is new and somewhat vague. It is difficult to know the dividing line between service quality and service value. Contributing to the difficulty in understanding exactly what is meant by "value" is the fact that not all stakeholders define quality and value in the same way. However, the following examples of the various definitions of service quality and service value may further the understanding of the difference between quality and value from the perspective of each stakeholder.

Client's Definition of Quality and Value

Quality is:

- knowing the extent to which therapy will help before treatment begins
- the greatest degree of symptom relief
- the best services for the least cost

Value is:

- responsiveness to client-identified needs and concerns
- timely provision of services
- the highest level of functional improvement
- the shortest possible duration of treatment
- a long-lasting outcome
- prevention of complications
- user-friendly communication

- the degree of concern expressed by the therapist
- the degree of courtesy exhibited by the therapist
- the convenience of the therapy (e.g., short transportation time, scheduled at the patient's convenience, easy access, etc.)
- no duplication of information requested by different departments and therapists
- a *total experience* that is highly satisfactory

Payer's Definition of Quality and Value

Quality is:

- the best outcome for the least cost
- outcome established before treatment begins
- length of treatment established before treatment begins
- timely provision of services
- timely transfer of patient to the most appropriate level of care
- outcomes that last over time

Value is:

- provider's demonstrated ability to control costs
- objectively demonstrated and good cost/benefit ratio
- prevention of complications related to the medical condition
- prevention of new and unrelated medical problems
- return to the highest possible level of productivity
- high customer satisfaction

Provider's Definition of Quality and Value

Quality is:

- the best outcome with the least consumption of resources
- the best outcome achieved with the least expensive resources

- outcomes predicted before treatment begins
- length of treatment established before treatment begins
- patient progress monitored and managed by critical pathways
- treatment provided on the basis of standardized treatment protocols
- the predicted outcome is achieved at or before the established length of treatment

Value is:

- high customer satisfaction
- outcomes achieved for the least cost
- rehabilitation practices and results that maintain existing and obtain new managed care contracts

While there are some differences in what all the stakeholders view as quality and value, there is a common thread that links all of them.

Quality is seen as:

- knowing the outcome prior to the commencement of treatment
- achieving that outcome at or before the expected time
- obtaining the highest level of functional improvement possible
- receiving treatment at the most appropriate place of care
- obtaining an outcome that lasts over time

Value is seen as:

- high satisfaction with the outcome of the services that were received
- a good cost/benefit outcome, meaning the highest functional outcome for the least cost, no recidivism after discharge, and low consumption of other health resources

Program Evaluation

The characteristics of value and quality described above can be expressed in what one might call the value equation of rehabilitation.

THE VALUE EQUATION

$$\frac{\text{Effectiveness}}{\text{Efficiency}} + \text{High Customer Satisfaction} = \text{Value}$$

To evaluate the rehabilitation program and test whether it has met the value equation, outcome studies must be conducted that address the following questions:

1. Has the outcome resulted in the client's increased ability to participate in life?
2. Has the best outcome been achieved for the least cost?
3. Is the outcome durable?
4. Is the client highly satisfied with the outcome?
5. Have the attained outcomes held down the overall cost of health care?

It is not enough simply to say the client got "better," that the client improved. Therapists must develop measures that clearly define what "better" is and develop measures of the cost effectiveness of getting "better."

Outcome Studies

The purpose of conducting outcome studies is to improve the quality of services provided by a rehabilitation program to a specific diagnostic group.[1] Such studies provide therapists, program managers, and administrators with a way to systematically evaluate the outcome of their rehabilitation efforts in relation to the: (1) appropriateness of the services rendered, (2) effectiveness of the services rendered, (3) adequacy with which they served the needs of their clients, and (4) effectiveness and efficiency of program management.[2]

Outcome studies evaluate the success of treatment in relation to previously established quality outcome indicators. The results of outcome studies help identify problem areas requiring more detailed investigation. Such detailed analysis determines whether treatment strategies or programs should be modified or whether completely new approaches should be instituted. The results of the detailed analysis may also help to refine appropriate level of care criteria, predict the expected outcomes for each level of care, refine the critical pathways utilized to produce those out-comes, and refine treatment protocols.[3]

Outcome study results also provide a basis for objective and informed decision making for future program planning, a database for research, and data to influence health care policy makers.[4]

What Should Outcome Studies Measure?

Historically, therapists have set long- and short-term goals and mea-sured progress toward them. Consequently, one might conclude that therapists are already measuring outcomes and, therefore, are already demonstrating treatment effectiveness. Goal attainment and therapy out-come, however, do not measure the same thing. Goals are related to the impairments that must be reduced or the abilities that must be attained upon completion of therapy. Long-term goals identify the ultimate destina-tion of therapy and short-term goals serve as the map for reaching that destination. The outcome (i.e., result) of therapy is what the client is able to do once the destination has been reached. The outcome of therapy, then, transcends the attainment of a certain level of independence in personal, household, and community activities of daily living (ADLs). The outcome of therapy is measured by the quality of life that one is able to live as a result of having achieved one's goals. Goal attainment measures the degree of progress a client makes as a result of therapy and the outcome measures the value or worth of that progress to the client, the client's family, the payer, and society in general.

Within this context, outcome studies must measure those aspects of rehabilitation services that will shed light on the following questions:

1. Do the services therapists provide reduce and/or compensate for disability?
2. Do these services result in a higher quality of life?
3. Which services are the least costly (e.g., produce the best results in the least amount of time with the least resource consumption)?
4. Do the outcomes attained by these services hold down the overall costs of health care (e.g., facilitate fast movement from a more intense level of care to a less intense level, prevent complications, prevent illness or conditions for which individuals are at high risk due to their impairments, and prevent recidivism)?

To provide data that respond to these questions, outcome studies should focus on the four key elements of service delivery: (1) effectiveness, (2) efficiency, (3) quality, and (4) value.

Effectiveness. Regarding this element of service delivery, outcome studies should be designed to determine which assessment procedures available for each diagnostic group most accurately and consistently identify and define that group's impairments and disabilities. They should also discover which treatment procedures available for each diagnostic group most consistently produce the expected increase in functional status.

Efficiency. Outcome studies should measure the array of assessment procedures available for each diagnostic group, in order to determine which ones take the least amount of time to accurately identify and define the impairments and disabilities of that group; which are absolutely necessary to identify and define that group's impairments and disabilities; which treatment procedures take the least amount of time to produce the expected increase in functional status; which of these treatment procedures that take the least amount of time are absolutely necessary to produce the expected increase in functional status; which ones produce an increase in functional status that is maintained over time without further therapeutic intervention; and which procedures available for each have the highest correlation with the best outcomes.

Quality. Outcome studies should measure aspects of a rehabilitation program that result in the provision of the most appropriate, effective, and efficient clinical services. Appropriate clinical services include assessment and treatment procedures that are the most specific and effective to the needs of a specific diagnostic group. Effective services are defined as those assessment and treatment procedures that have the highest correlation with the greatest functional gains. Efficient clinical services are those assessment and treatment procedures that have the highest correlation with both the greatest functional gains and the least frequency, intensity, and duration of treatment, as well as the greatest durability.

Value. Outcome studies should measure the value of rehabilitation services in the following terms: Do the gains in function that result from clinical services also result in greater ability of the individuals of a diagnostic group to participate in life? Do the gains in function that result from clinical services also result in high customer satisfaction? Do the gains in function that result from clinical services also hold down overall costs (e.g., prevent illness or conditions for which patients are at higher risk due to their impairments/disabilities, contribute to reducing length of stay, prevent rehospitalization, reduce collateral caregiver costs, etc.)?

Types of Outcome Studies

There are three types of outcome studies: (1) rehabilitation outcome studies, (2) customer satisfaction outcome studies, and (3) financial outcome studies.

Rehabilitation Outcome Studies

Rehabilitation outcome studies evaluate whether the clients served in a rehabilitation program achieved the skills and abilities that the team predicted and, if so, whether those skills and abilities were maintained after discharge from rehabilitation and whether they resulted in an enhanced quality of life. Rehabilitation outcome studies employ measurement instruments that are designed to measure the degree of improvement in functional status between admission and discharge from a rehabilitation program and to measure the degree to which clients sustained their discharge level of function after discharge. Rehabilitation studies also use instruments that are designed to measure the client's perceived quality of life after discharge from the rehabilitation program.

Example Functional Improvement Instruments

FIM™ Instrument*
The FIM instrument is an 18-item, 7-level scale that assesses severity of disability and generates a profile of an individual's ability to perform daily living tasks related to each of the above noted measurement domains.[5] Scores for each of the 18 items may be summed to generate a total FIM score. Also, FIM scores can be broken out into a motor FIM score and a cognitive FIM score. It is administered by any person who undergoes

---

* Functional Independence Measure. Copyright © 1996, Uniform Data System for Medical Rehabilitation, a division of UB Foundation Activities, Inc.

training. Training may include self-study of the FIM *Guide*, review of training videos, or participation in a training workshop. The FIM instrument is administered within 72 hours of admission and discharge. Follow-up assessments are usually obtained by a telephone interview 80 to 180 days after discharge from rehabilitation. The results of the FIM instrument or evaluation can also be used to provide data regarding the cost-effectiveness of rehabilitation when they are analyzed in relation to length of stay and amount of therapy provided during that length of stay.[6]

The FIM instrument is the most widely used outcome measurement tool. It is used is by the Uniform Data System for Medical Rehabilitation (UDSMR) to provide subscribing rehabilitation facilities with outcome information for each diagnostic category they serve, as well as information that allows providers to compare their outcomes, regionally and nationally, with other rehabilitation facilities' outcomes.

- Target population: Persons seven years of age or older who sustained a stroke, brain injury, orthopedic impairments, spinal cord dysfunction, arthritis, or debility. It has also been used with persons with cancer and acquired immune deficiency syndrome.
- Measurement domains:
  1. self-care
  2. sphincter control
  3. transfers
  4. communication
  5. social cognition

Functional Assessment Measure (FAM)[7]

The FAM is similar in intent and format to the FIM instrument. It consists of the 18 items found in the FIM instrument, but incorporates 12 additional items related to cognitive and behavioral functions, communication, and community.

- Target population: Stroke and traumatic brain injury (can be used for all disabilities)
- Measurement domains: Same as FIM instrument with 12 additional items in the domains noted above.
- Administration time: Approximately 35 minutes. It can be administered by clinical observation, in a patient conference, or by telephone.

- Administration procedure: Same as the FIM instrument

Patient Evaluation Conference System (PECS)[8]

- Target population: All disability groups
- Measurement domains: Functions related to:
  1. rehabilitation medicine
  2. rehabilitation nursing
  3. pulmonary rehabilitation
  4. medications
  5. nutrition
  6. mobility
  7. activities of daily living
  8. assistive devices
  9. communication
  10. psychology
  11. social functioning
  12. educational functioning
  13. leisure activity
  14. pastoral care
- Administration time: The PECS is composed of 93 items and is quite comprehensive. Depending upon team members' level of training in its use and/or client complexity, it can take 45 minutes to 1 hour to complete.
- Administration procedure: Assessment items are assigned to disciplines. At the time of admission, each discipline rates the client's current level of function, using a scale of 0–7 for each assigned measurement domain and establishes the goal discharge level of function using the same 0–7 scale. The client is then measured in the same manner at the time of discharge. Because of its length, follow-up administrations are usually not performed unless the client returns to the rehabilitation facility for that purpose.

Levels of Rehabilitation Scale (LORS)[9]

- Target population: The LORS was utilized on a stroke population but could be used with other neurologic impairment groups.
- Measurement domains: Activities of daily living, cognition, home activities, outside-of-home activities, social interaction, and vocational status

- Administration time: 5 to 10 minutes
- Administration procedure: One person who is very familiar with the client (usually a nurse) rates the client, using a 5-point scale, on each of the 47 assessment items at the time of admission, at discharge, and at six-week and four-and-a-half-month follow-ups. The home and outside-the-home activities, as well as the social interaction items, also provide some measurement of degree of handicap.

Rehabilitation Institute of Chicago Functional Assessment Scale (RICFAS)[10]
The RICFAS* is composed of 18 items from the FIM and 37 additional items that are designed to measure a broader range of skills than found in the FIM. For example, the RICFAS provides a more in-depth assessment of communication, psychosocial, vocational, and leisure skills.

- Target population: All rehabilitation diagnoses
- Measurement domains:
  1. medical management
  2. health maintenance
  3. self-care
  4. mobility
  5. communication
  6. cognition
  7. psychosocial
  8. community integration
- Administration time: 35 minutes.
- Administration procedure: The RICFAS is administered by designated disciplines and scored in the same manner as the FIM.

Disability Rating Scale (DRS)[11]

- Target population: Traumatic brain injury
- Measurement domains: Level of arousal/awareness, cognitive ability, physical dependence, and adaptability for work
- Administration time: 5 to 10 minutes

Source: Reprinted with permission from Rehabilitation Institute of Chicago, *Functional Assessment Scale Version IV,* © 1996.

- Administration procedure: Administered by one person at the time of admission and discharge. Can be used for either telephone or in-person follow-up interview. It has the ability to track changes in an individual from coma to community living on a set of global measurement domains.

The quality of life measurement instruments highlighted below include the following: the Community Integration Questionnaire, the Craig Handicap Assessment and Reporting Technique, the Medical Rehabilitation Follow Along Instrument, the Short Form-36, the Sickness Impact Profile, and the Life Satisfaction Index-A.

Community Integration Questionnaire (CIQ)[12]

- Target population: Traumatic brain injury; can also be used with other disability groups since it measures abilities that are common to all disability groups
- Measurement domains:
  1. household activities
  2. shopping
  3. errands
  4. leisure activities
  5. visiting friends
  6. social events
  7. performance of productive activities
- Administration time: 10 to 15 minutes
- Administration procedure: It can be self-administered or administered by personal interview or by telephone. It is typically administered at discharge and at periodic follow-up intervals.

Craig Handicap Assessment and Reporting Technique (CHART)[13]

- Target population: Spinal cord injury
- Measurement domains:
  1. physical independence
  2. mobility
  3. social integration
  4. occupation
  5. economics
- Administration time: 15 minutes

- Administration procedure: The CHART is designed as an interview instrument. It can be administered either face to face or by telephone. It can also be mailed to the client. However, as the authors point out, valuable data may be lost when the instrument is mailed because of the absence of an interaction between the interviewer and the client. It is recommended that it be administered multiple times over the course of the client's lifetime after discharge from rehabilitation.

Medical Rehabilitation Follow Along Instrument (MRFA)[14]*

- Target population: All disability groups. The MRFA is designed for medical rehabilitation outpatient settings.
- Measurement domains: Physical functioning, pain experience, effective well-being, and cognitive functioning; these areas of assessment measure the quality of daily living of persons with disability. The MRFA has three different formats: musculoskeletal, neurologic, and multiple sclerosis.
- Administration time: 20 to 30 minutes
- Administration procedures: The client report components of the MRFA may be self-administered or conducted with an interview format. The neurologic form is administered by the clinician through an interview with the client and caregiver. The multiple sclerosis form is administered by the client's clinician.

Short Form-36 (SF-36).[15] The SF-36 was developed to measure a patient's perception of wellness. It consists of 36 questions that are designed to measure the following eight areas of health:

- physical functioning
- role limitations due to physical health
- role limitations due to emotional problems
- energy/fatigue
- emotional well-being
- social functioning
- pain
- general health

Source: Reprinted with permission from C. Granger et al., Reliability of a Brief Outpatient Functional Outcome Assessment Measure, *American Journal of Physical Medicine and Rehabilitation*, Vol. 74, No. 6, pp. 469–475, © 1995, Williams & Wilkins.

Sickness Impact Profile (SIP68).[16] The SIP68 contains 68 questions and is divided into the following six subscales:*

1. somatic autonomy
2. mobility control
3. psychic autonomy and communication
4. social behavior
5. emotional stability
6. mobility range

Life Satisfaction Index-A.[17] This instrument addresses the following 12 daily living domains:*

1. family relationships
2. spiritual life
3. daily living tasks
4. housing
5. transportation
6. emotional well-being
7. general health
8. social life
9. recreational life
10. money matters
11. sex life
12. employment

Customer Satisfaction Outcome Studies

Therapists typically focus on providing the best treatment possible and therefore expect that the client's degree of satisfaction will be strongly related to their knowledge, technical skill, and the degree to which the client's impairments and disabilities are relieved as a result of their professional skills. While technical knowledge, skills, and judgment are most definitely linked to customer satisfaction, they are far from the only variables that create a satisfactory or unsatisfactory rehabilitation experience.

Source: Reprinted with permission of the Gerontological Society of America, 1030 15th Street, NW, Suite 250, Washington, DC 20005. The Measurement of Life Satisfaction, B. Neugarten et al., *Journal of Gerontology,* 1961, Vol. 16. Reproduced by permission of the publisher via Copyright Clearance Center, Inc.

Client satisfaction or dissatisfaction is a complicated phenomenon that is linked to the client's expectations, health status, and personal characteristics, as well as to the characteristics of the health care system providing the service.[18] It is based on the client's subjective experiences, his or her expectations and behavior as a participant in the treatment process, as well as on the perceived technical quality and service quality provided by the service provider. Customer satisfaction is based on the client's total experience of the rehabilitation encounter, not its individual components. Understanding clients' experience of rehabilitation requires an understanding of how they perceive their needs. Clients' perception of their needs will dictate their expectations of the rehabilitation experience. Although customer satisfaction is based on the client's subjective evaluation of the total experience and is highly individualistic, the Picker Institute has identified eight dimensions of care that are especially critical to a satisfactory experience from the client's point of view:*

1. Access: Clients are negatively affected by barriers to accessing health care such as telephone triage or voice mail systems, travel distance, scheduling difficulties, and restrictions imposed by payers.
2. Respect: Clients have a strong need to be recognized and treated with dignity and respect as individuals. A sense of anonymity can lead to a sense of a loss of identity within the context of the rehabilitation process. It is the sense of lost identity that creates the feelings of not being treated with respect. Clients also judge respect on the basis of the degree to which the therapists inform and involve them in treatment decisions. Regardless of how therapeutically respectful a therapist is, the client who feels like just one more widget or feels left out of decisions about his or her care will have a negative total experience.
3. Coordination: The client's perception of the therapist's competency and efficiency are shaped by how well all aspects of the rehabilitation process are coordinated.
4. Information, communication, and education: Clients have a strong need to feel informed about their clinical status, progress, and prognosis; informed about the process of rehabilitation; and informed about ways of managing on their own when they are discharged. Informed in this context does not simply mean that they have been told something about their care; instead, they must feel knowledgeable,

---

Source: Reprinted with permission from *A Report from The American Hospital Association and The Picker Institute*, pp. 1–13, © 1997, American Hospital Association and The Picker Institute.

confident, and competent as a result of the information they have received. Clients who fear that information is being withheld from them, that they are not being completely or honestly informed about their condition or prognosis, or those who actually have such experiences, will be very dissatisfied with their rehabilitation experience regardless of the quality of the actual outcome.

5. Physical comfort: Clients view physical care that comforts them as one of the most elemental services a caregiver can provide. Clean, comfortable, and pleasant surroundings are also perceived as part of the desired physical comfort.

6. Emotional support: While clients do not readily express their anxieties and fears, their need for emotional support is nonetheless paramount. They need support in dealing not only with their anxiety about their illness and its outcome but also with its affect on their ability to care for themselves and those that depend upon them, as well as concerns about the cost of care and its impact on the current and long-term well-being of their family.

7. Involvement of family and friends: Family members and close friends can provide social and emotional support. They also often function as proxy decision makers when the client is unable to participate in decision making. Often family or friends are the primary caregivers after the client is discharged from rehabilitation. While the clients must rely on their family and friends for these types of assistance, they simultaneously worry about the impact of their illness on their caregivers.

8. Transition and continuity: Clients often experience a discontinuity of care as they move across the inpatient, home care, and outpatient levels of care. Their lack of understanding of the institutional and functional boundaries of the various levels of care make it difficult to effectively negotiate the transition from one level of care to another.

It is quite noticeable that technical skills and their effectiveness are not listed in the eight dimensions of care linked to customer satisfaction or dissatisfaction. Most assuredly, clients do expect to improve as a result of rehabilitation and the lack thereof will definitely influence their perceived satisfaction with it. The nature of the eight dimensions that influence client satisfaction, as identified by the Picker Institute, however, indicate that satisfaction is more greatly influenced by how rehabilitation services are provided than by their technical proficiency.

The methods used to gather customer satisfaction information varies among providers from comment cards, mail surveys, in-person interviews, telephone interviews, and focus groups. Some providers also seek their employees' perceptions of the quality of service provision. Work teams, quality circles, and focus groups are several methods used to identify service delivery problems and recommended solutions. Regardless of the method used to gather customer satisfaction data, it is extremely important that the instrument used contains questions that are designed to measure clients' experiences in the eight dimensions of care identified by the Picker Institute, as well as questions related to the technical quality and outcome of the care that has been rendered. It is also important to measure customer satisfaction during the course of rehabilitation as well as after discharge. By measuring it during rehabilitation, problems can be immediately identified and rectified and, therefore, a potentially unsatisfactory experience can be averted.

Financial Outcome Studies

Financial outcome studies measure the cost/benefit ratio of the services that have been provided. These studies analyze three questions: (1) What was the degree of improvement in relation to the dollars spent to achieve it? (2) Did the improvement make a difference? and (3) Which treatment approaches are the most effective and least expensive?

Regarding the relationship of dollars spent to the degree of improvement, the basic question is, "What is the relationship between the degree of functional gain and the number of therapy units of service expended to achieve it?" To answer this question, one must collect data regarding the types of therapy units provided, the number of each type that was provided, and the outcome that was produced. The FIM instrument, described earlier, is one of the most widely used cost/benefit measurement instruments. Many providers contract with the Uniform Data System for Medical Rehabilitation (UDSmr) to provide them with a "performance report" on a quarterly basis. This report is based on FIM change score, length of stay, and charge data that providers submit to the UDSmr on a monthly basis. Each quarter or annually, providers receive a report regarding six performance indicators: (1) length of stay by impairment group, (2) change in total FIM score from admission and discharge, (3) length of stay efficiency, (4) change in FIM per week, (5) charge efficiency, and (6) discharge destination and Program Evaluation Performance Index. The performance report also provides data that allow providers to compare their performance with other providers, both regionally and nationally. Of these six performance indicators, the length of stay (LOS) efficiency and charge efficiency indicators provide the cost/benefit information. Since clients utilize rehabilitation services and facilities on a daily basis, a client's length of stay is a measurement of the cost of rehabilitation, i.e., the longer the length of stay, the greater the cost. The LOS efficiency is calculated by subtracting the admission FIM score from the discharge FIM score and dividing the difference (the amount of functional gain by the client's length of stay in days. The most efficient (i.e., least costly) outcome with the highest benefit to the client is the one in which the highest FIM score difference is achieved in the shortest period of time. Service charges are also used as another cost/benefit measure. Charge efficiency is calculated by subtracting the client's admission FIM from the discharge FIM and dividing the difference (the amount of functional gain) by charges (in dollars) for services provided to that client and then multiplying that number by 1,000. Charge efficiency, then, is expressed by the amount of FIM gain per $1,000 charged. Again, as with LOS efficiency, the best outcome from a cost/benefit perspective is where the highest FIM score difference is attained for the least charges. Changes, however, are very rough estimates of costs. As providers develop actual cost data, they will be able to calculate the true cost efficiency of an outcome.

For example, one could compare the number of FIM units gained in each functional area of the FIM or the amount of change in the total FIM score from admission to discharge with the number of hours of treatment expended. From this comparison, one could create a ratio between the number of FIM units gained per hour of treatment expended. From a financial perspective, a good outcome would be one in which a high number of FIM units are gained in relation to a low number of therapy units (dollars) expended. Clearly a bad outcome would be one in which the number of FIM units gained is low and the expended therapy hours is high.

Which treatment approaches produce the best cost to benefit ratio? There is wide variation among practitioners with respect to treatment approaches utilized for a particular diagnostic population and individuals within that population. It cannot be assumed that all are equally efficient and effective. Consequently, it is not enough to look only at the number of therapy units provided. The type of therapy units must also be analyzed to determine which treatment approaches produce the greatest improvement for the least cost.

Life Satisfaction

The third component of the cost/benefit analysis relates to the degree to which rehabilitation outcomes make a difference in the lives of those who received the services. Here, one would examine the relationship between the number and type of therapy units expended and an individual's ability to perform in real-life situations, whether the gains made in rehabilitation are sustained or even improved across time after discharge, and whether life satisfaction is higher after discharge.

CONCLUSION

As discussed in Chapter 2, a prospective payment system (PPS) requires that providers manage their costs in order to make a profit. Prior to the PPS reimbursement model, providers simply reduced staff when they experienced a decline in their profit margins. In these, the beginning phases of capitated reimbursement, management's response has not only been staff reductions, but also to move in the direction of less costly aide-delivered services and services delivered in a group therapy format rather than individual therapy. This very simplistic, yet effective, short-term approach to cost management will predictably lead to decreased quality of care. Decreased quality of care, in turn, will just as predictably lead to decreased profitability. If quality declines, providers will lose existing contracts with managed care organizations and will be unable to negotiate new contracts with other managed care organizations. Managed care organizations will contract with those providers who not only control their costs, but are able to do so while maintaining quality of care. In some instances, staff reductions may be reasonable and can be accomplished without compromising quality of care. Similarly, it cannot be argued that the use of aides and group therapy automatically means poor quality of care. Quality will not suffer if aide-delivered services and group therapy are employed on the basis of well-reasoned clinical criteria and guidelines. However, even when appropriately employed, these three approaches to cost management will not be sufficient to ensure good quality of care and profitability in a managed care environment. For, as Burgess has pointed out, "When health care professionals continue to operate via old protocols, procedures, and priorities within a new practice paradigm, the achievement of quality outcomes within the client's benefit package is difficult, if not impossible."[19] To manage costs and simultaneously produce quality outcomes, providers must redesign their service delivery systems. The production of the best outcome for the least cost will require a service delivery process that is well choreographed, tightly focused, continually monitored, and coordinated, as well as continually self-improving. The MORsystem provides a framework within which to redesign a provider's service delivery system. Chapter 3 identified the components of the service delivery process that the team is to manage. The client management plan presented in Chapter 4 provides the choreography required to manage those components. The rehabilitation process management system presented in this chapter provides a method of creating a tightly focused (prospective management), continually monitored and coordinated (concurrent management), and self-improving (retrospective management) service delivery system. The central feature of prospective and concurrent management is the assurance of the medical necessity of services. These two management systems guide the team through the clinical decision-making process that ensures that the services that they are about to provide are reasonable and necessary to the client's condition, that the client is making significant practical improvement throughout the entire course of rehabilitation, that nonskilled services are provided at the appropriate time, and that the services are being provided at the appropriate level of care. Retrospective clinical case management (i.e., outcome studies) acts to ensure the continual improvements of the appropriateness, effectiveness, efficiency, and value of the provided services.

REFERENCES

1. S. Forer, How To Make Program Evaluation Work for You, *NeuroRehabilitation 2*, no. 4 (1992): 52–71.
2. S. Forer, "Outcome Analysis for Program Service Management," in *Rehabilitation Outcomes: Analysis and Measurement*, ed. M. Fuhrer (Baltimore: Paul H. Brookes Publishing, 1987), 187–203.
3. R. Carey and E. Posavac, Rehabilitation Program Evaluation Using a Revised Level of Rehabilitation Scale, *Archives of Physical Medicine and Rehabilitation 63* (1982): 367–370.
4. S. Forer, How To Make Program Evaluation Work for You, 52–71.
5. State University of New York at Buffalo, Research Foundation, *Guide for Use of the Uniform Data System for Medical Rehabilitation: Functional Independence Measure* (Buffalo: 1990).

6. B. Hamilton et al., A Uniform National Data System for Medical Rehabilitation," in *Rehabilitation Outcomes: Analysis and Measurement*, ed. M. Furher (Baltimore: Paul H. Brookes Publishing, 1987), 137.

7. K. Hall et al., Functional Measures after Traumatic Brain Injury: Ceiling Effects of FIM, FIM + FAM, DRS, and CIQ, *Journal of Head Trauma Rehabilitation 11*, no. 5 (1996): 27–39.

8. H. Richard and H. Jellinek, Functional Performance Assessment: A Program Approach, *Archives of Physical Medicine and Rehabilitation 62* (1981): 456–460.

9. Carey and Posavac, "Rehabilitation Program Evaluation."

10. Rehabilitation Institute of Chicago, *Functional Assessment Scale Version IV* (Chicago: 1996).

11. M. Rappaport et al., Disability Rating Scale for Severe Head Trauma: Coma to Community, *Archives of Physical Medicine and Rehabilitation 63* (1982): 118–123.

12. B. Willer et al., Community Integration following Rehabilitation for Traumatic Brain Injury, *Journal of Head Trauma Rehabilitation 8*, no. 2 (1993): 75–87.

13. G. Whiteneck et al., Quantifying Handicap: A New Measure of Long-Term Outcomes, *Archives of Physical Medicine and Rehabilitation 73* (1992): 519–525.

14. C. Granger et al., Reliability of a Brief Outpatient Functional Outcome Assessment Measure, *American Journal of Physical Medicine and Rehabilitation 74*, no. 6 (1995): 469–475.

15. C.A. McHorney et al., The MOS 36-Item Short-Form Health Survey (SF-36): Psychometric and Clinical Tests of Validity in Measuring Physical and Mental Health Constructs, *Medical Care 31* (1993): 247–263.

16. M. Bergner et al., Sickness Impact Profile: Development and Final Revision of a Health Status Measure, *Medical Care 8* (1981): 787–805.

17. B. Neugarten et al., The Measurement of Life Satisfaction, *Journal of Gerontology 16* (1961): 134–143.

18. M. Hseik and J. Kagle, Understanding Patient Satisfaction and Dissatisfaction with Health Care, *National Association of Social Workers 16* (1991): 281–290.

19. C. Burgess, Hitting the Wall, *Rehabilitation Management 13*, no. 6 (1996): 25–27.

CHAPTER 6

Family Management Tools

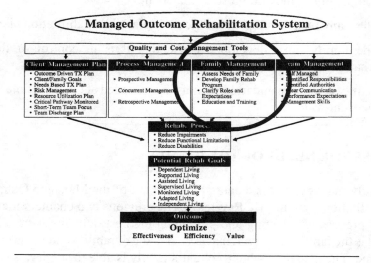

Managed Outcome Rehabilitation System

Quality and Cost Management Tools

Client Management Plan
- Outcome Driven TX Plan
- Client/Family Goals
- Needs Based TX Plan
- Risk Management
- Resource Utilization Plan
- Critical Pathway Monitored
- Short-Term Team Focus
- Team Discharge Plan

Process Management
- Prospective Management
- Concurrent Management
- Retrospective Management

Family Management
- Assess Needs of Family
- Develop Family Rehab Program
- Clarify Roles and Expectations
- Education and Training

Team Management
- Self Managed
- Identified Responsibilities
- Identified Authorities
- Clear Communication
- Performance Expectations
- Management Skills

Rehab. Process
- Reduce Impairments
- Reduce Functional Limitations
- Reduce Disabilities

Potential Rehab Goals
- Dependent Living
- Supported Living
- Assisted Living
- Supervised Living
- Monitored Living
- Adapted Living
- Independent Living

Outcome
Optimize
Effectiveness   Efficiency   Value

Family Management
- Assess Needs of Family
- Develop Family Rehab Program
- Clarify Roles and Expectations
- Provide Education and Training

KEY POINTS

- The family is equally as "injured" as the client.

- The rehabilitation team must treat the family as a unit, not just the client.

- The team must identify family impairments and disabilities as completely as they do those of the client.

- The team must develop and implement a family rehabilitation plan.

- The family must develop a sense that it is in control of the rehabilitation process.

- Family education and training must be provided at the right time in the right way.

ASSESS THE NEEDS OF THE FAMILY

Family management is a central component of the Managed Outcome Rehabilitation System (MORsystem). The previous two chapters focused on the process of selecting and producing the best outcome for the least cost. It is the family, however, that is vital to the durability and value of that outcome. The degree to which a client's family is able to support, sustain, and enhance his or her outcome after discharge from rehabilitation will be proportional to three factors: (1) the degree to which the family understands the purpose and process of rehabilitation, (2) the degree to which the family accepts the purpose and process of rehabilitation, and (3) the degree to which the family's impairments and disabilities, caused by the disruptive impact of the medical episode on the family unit, have been resolved. To facilitate a family unit that has the knowledge, skills, and emotional stamina required to support, sustain, and enhance the client's outcome, the team must establish and implement a family management plan that is as family-specific and vigorous as the client's management plan.

The Family Is the "Patient"

From both a quality and a cost management perspective, the family as a unit, not solely the client, is the focal point of rehabilitation. The client's rate of recovery and the durability of the achieved rehabilitation outcome will be significantly affected, either positively or negatively, by the degree to which family members understand and accept the client's impairments and disabilities and the degree to which they accept the changes that these disabilities have brought to the family unit. The family's ability and willingness to deal with these new realities is strongly correlated to family members' acceptance of and competence in their new roles and responsibilities. Such understanding and acceptance will result in family members who are better equipped to provide the emotional and practical support that the client needs, both during and after rehabilitation.

Treating the family as a unit is the key to a successful rehabilitation outcome. A medical episode that results in a disabling condition has a catastrophic impact on both the individual who experiences it as well as the individual's family. The client is devastated by the diminished or lost skills and abilities that now significantly alter his or her role in the family, and the family is equally as devastated by the effects of these losses on them. Both parties are disabled but in different ways. The client's disabilities are tied to observable physical impairments. Family disabilities, on the other hand, are not as visible. They do not emanate from impaired physical structures and body systems; instead they occur in areas such as loss or alteration of relationships, changes in roles and responsibilities, loss of a sense of control over their lives, emotional turmoil, doubts about their future, loss of financial stability, and disruption in their ability to carry out their typical daily living routines. Both the client and members of the client's family are injured and both require rehabilitation. The client is part of an interactive and interdependent family unit. The alteration of the skills, abilities, and roles of one member of that unit reciprocally alters, in some way, the skills, abilities, and roles of all other members of that unit. Consequently, the client cannot be taken out of the family unit, treated, and returned to it on the presumption that the family unit can independently and effectively reconstitute itself in a manner that will both support the achieved outcome and simultaneously meet the needs of all other family members.

Family Response to Disablement

From the moment of the acute medical episode through the eventual discharge from rehabilitation, the family begins a journey that will take them through many phases of "family disability." While each phase has its unique characteristics, there will be a common theme underlying all of them. Prior to the medical episode, all members of the family unit, individually and as a whole, had a sense of predictability and, therefore, control over their lives. The needs, goals, and aspirations of each family member were known and the family unit had established patterns of responsibilities and interaction that, for better or worse, functioned predictably to meet each other's needs and support each other's goals and aspirations. All family members felt in charge of and in control of their lives. When a medical episode afflicts one family member, the sense of predictability and control over one's life is shattered. The family unit is thrown out of balance. Each member, including the client, experiences a loss of control over their lives. It is the family's desire and struggle to regain balance and control that permeates all phases of rehabilitation.

The family's need and desire to regain control is a natural response to the loss of predictability and control. They had no control over the occurrence of the medical episode nor of the immediate and drastic changes it brought into their lives. They are thrust into a situation that is occurring in an unfamiliar environment and they have no experiential framework within which to understand what is happening to them and their injured family member. They feel they have no control over the rehabilitation process nor its outcome and they are faced with terminology that is foreign, long-term care planning as well as financial and, sometimes, legal issues. During the acute medical intervention phase the family gradually learned the caregiving process, its procedures, as well as the personalities of the caregivers and how to deal with them. They may have even begun to trust and bond with certain members of the staff. In essence, they began to have a sense of predictability and control over their lives, but they find that it has to be regained again and again each time the client is discharged to a subsequent level of care.

The need and desire to regain control and predictability is the ever-present quest of the family unit as it progresses through the response to disablement, which occurs in the following stages: shock and disbelief, elation and joy, reality, and crisis and despair.[1] (See Exhibit 6–1.)

Just as rehabilitation does not "cure" the client's impairments, so too family rehabilitation does not obviate the family's journey through the phases of response to disablement. Both the client's and the family's rehabilitation programs provide the knowledge, insight, tools, and strategies that will enable them to compensate for and cope with their respective

Exhibit 6–1 Phases of Family Response to Disablement

Shock and disbelief
Client's medical crisis is the focus of the family; family experiences feelings of helplessness and depends heavily on medical personnel for information and decision making.

Elation and joy
Medical crisis is over; there is hope for recovery; family does not grasp the potential for long-term disability and its impact on the family unit, nor do they seriously consider it when presented by medical staff.

Reality
Increased awareness of the permanency of the loss sustained; feelings of loss begin to emerge as do questions from the family such as: How and why could this event occur? Why has it resulted in possible long-term disability? What will be the eventual type and degree of disability? and What will our life be like in the future?

Crisis and despair
Grief and anxiety emerge as the family faces the future and begins to mourn its losses; comprehension of information provided to them is impaired and problem solving is difficult; they require considerable support simply to survive the moment and the grieving process as it begins.

Source: Reprinted from K. Hall et al., Functional Measures after Traumatic Brain Injury: Ceiling Effects of FIM, FIM & FAM, DRS, and CIQ, *Journal of Head Trauma Rehabilitation*, Vol. 11, no. 5, pp. 27–39, 1996, Aspen Publishers.

---

disabilities. While family members are experiencing different kinds of disabilities, their degree of disability is determined in the same way as the client's. It is determined by the degree to which a gap exists between the family's abilities and the demands of the environments within which they are called upon to function. Family rehabilitation, therefore, focuses on identifying the type and nature of the gaps between the family's existing abilities and demands of their environments and implementing a treatment plan designed to provide them with the tools to bridge the gaps.

The Goal of Family Rehabilitation

The goal of a family rehabilitation program is to avoid client regression after discharge from rehabilitation. Codependency is the primary cause of regression from an achieved level of independence. Codependency is a two-way process between the client and a family member or the family as a whole and can manifest in one of two ways. It may emanate from the client in the form of asking for or demanding that family members do for the client that which the client is capable of doing and the family acquiescing to these demands. Or it may emanate from family members either in the form of overhelping or underhelping. The goal of the family rehabilitation program, then, is to facilitate the right level of helping. "Right helping" is the provision of the right type and amount of support in the right manner and at the right time and place. The right level of helping bridges the gap between the client's abilities and the demands of the environment. Right helping facilitates the reconstitution of the family unit around a new set of family roles, rules, and responsibilities and helps facilitate the return of balance to the family unit.

The objective of a family rehabilitation program is to facilitate the family unit's ability to regain a sense of predictability and control over their lives, a sense of knowing their future, and being in charge of it. The family rehabilitation program works toward the following goals:

- Facilitate active involvement of the client's family in the rehabilitation process.
- Facilitate family understanding of and adaptation to the effects of the client's disabilities on the family system.
- Provide the family with the emotional and practical tools required to sustain the client's outcome after discharge.

A family rehabilitation program is based on the following suppositions:

- The family wants its loved one to recover as fully as possible and to be as independent as possible.
- The family has never had to deal with a disabled family member before.
- Family members want to help but are not sure how best to support their loved one's progress.
- Family members care enough to learn how best to help their loved one.
- Family members care enough to learn how to keep the family unit functioning in a healthy manner (i.e., to avoid codependency).

DEVELOP A FAMILY REHAB PROGRAM

The family rehabilitation program is based on an assessment of the family's needs and the development and implementation of a family treatment plan based on the results of the assessment.

Assessment

Just as there is no one-size-fits-all client treatment plan, there is no a generic approach to family rehabilitation. The purpose of a family assessment is to develop an individualized family rehabilitation plan. The family assessment identifies specific areas of family disability that must be treated to develop the skills and coping strategies that will allow family members to respond successfully to the demands of the environments within which they and the client will function.

Identify General Level of Functioning

The family's general level of functioning must be established first. To be successful, all intervention strategies and techniques must be commensurate with the family member's current ability to intellectually, emotionally, and motivationally engage in, learn, retain, and employ those strategies and techniques.

The rehabilitation team's first task is to identify the phase of family reaction to disablement (Exhibit 6–1). All members of the team can assist in determining whether the family is in the shock and disbelief, elation and joy, reality, or crisis and despair phase by reporting their behavioral observations at team conferences. Some family members may require an interview with a social worker or psychologist. The team should bear in mind that it is also possible that different family members may be in different phases during the same time period.

The team's next step in assessing family needs is to identify its stages of grieving. The stages of grieving were first defined by Elisabeth Kubler-Ross and are presented in Exhibit 6–2 along with behavioral examples of each stage drawn from the rehabilitation experience.[2] Typically, the family member's stage of grieving is established by the social worker and/or psychologist on the team. The day-to-day observations of all team mem-

Exhibit 6–2 Stages of Grief

Shock: Feelings of numbness and being easily overwhelmed. At this stage, the family has extreme difficulty processing, understanding information, and retaining it. Everything is a blur. There may be expressions of hopelessness and helplessness.

Denial: At this stage, the family has difficulty accepting the whole picture, focuses on a small part of the problem, does not acknowledge the painful aspects of what has happened, and focuses only on those changes in the client that provide them with signs of hope.

Anger: A family member at this stage may express anger over why this has happened to the family and the client. There may be anger directed at staff for perceived inadequate or inappropriate care. The family member may not be supportive of the team's efforts by either overhelping or underhelping. This individual may have fragmented and distorted recall of staff-provided information, which results in inappropriate or inaccurate helping and the constant seeking of clarification of the information from team members while simultaneously blaming them for not providing the answers to his or her questions.

Bargaining: The family member may feel some level of responsibility (guilt) for the client's medical condition (e.g., "If only I was home when it happened," "If we hadn't argued before he left for work," or "If I had only made him stick to what his doctor told him to do."). On the other hand, they may not feel a sense of responsibility but believe that if they offer to do something better or different now or in the future, then the appealed higher power (God, therapists, physicians) will make the client better.

Depression: Depression emerges when the family members begin to acknowledge both that the client will have some level of chronic disability and that this disability will affect the family unit. Family members may show signs of sadness or helplessness. Some members who were previously very involved in the client's program may withdraw while others may become overinvolved. Family members who in the past were calm and pleasant with the staff may become irritable and angered by seemingly minor things. Some family members may communicate that they are very fatigued, can't sleep well, don't feel like eating, and/or don't know if they can continue to cope with the situation.

Acceptance: This encompasses the movement from curing the disabled person so he or she will enjoy a full recovery to acceptance of the person's disabilities and the alterations they have brought to the family unit. It signals a change in the perception from "our family member is a disabled person" to "our family member is a person with a disability."

bers, however, are essential to confirming the social worker's/psychologist's opinion.

Identify Family Understanding of Disability

The rehabilitation team's next task is to rank or rate family members' degree of understanding of the nature and implications of the client's impairments and disabilities.[3] The Family Understanding of Disability Scale shown in Exhibit 6–3 is an example of a tool that the social worker or psychologist can use to perform this task. This scale can also be used to rate attitudes of family members toward disability and their perception of the client's future limits as a result of disability. The levels of understanding are ranked in order of 1–7 in the scale—7 signifying no problems dealing with the disability process, and 1 indicating severe problems comprehending the nature of the situation.

Identify Level of Family Adaptation

The team next wants to determine how well the family is adapting to the client's disabilities or impairments. The Family Adaptation Scale shown in Exhibit 6–4 is an example of a tool the social worker or psychologist can use to identify the family's adjustment to disability (i.e., their coping resources).[4]

Identify the Amount of Family Support Needed

The Support Network Scale shown in Exhibit 6–5 is an example of an assessment instrument that a social worker can use to identify the amount of assistance that the family will need in order to provide the required level of client care support both during rehabilitation and after discharge.[5]

A more in-depth family assessment may be required to gain the insight needed to assist those families who are judged to be functioning at levels 2, 3, and 4. An instrument such as the Family Assessment Device will be useful in this regard.[6] This is a 60-item self-administered questionnaire. It provides information regarding family problem solving, communication, roles, effective involvement, behavioral control, and general functioning.

Identify Family Needs

Family members often need help sorting out exactly what they need in order to cope with, participate in, and support the rehabilitation process. A

Exhibit 6–3 Family Understanding of Disability Scale

Includes the family's understanding of the nature and implications of illness/disability, including prognosis. Also includes family's receptivity to educational interventions.

Scale Points	Level	Behavioral Definition
7	No Problem	Complete understanding of disability and future implications.
6	Minimal Problem	Workable understanding of disability; open to further education.
5	Mild Problem	Workable understanding of disability; need moderate educational intervention.
4	Mild to Moderate Problem	Workable understanding; need maximal educational intervention.
3	Moderate Problem	Incomplete understanding; lack insight into educational needs.
2	Moderate to Severe Problem	Poor understanding; lack insight into educational needs.
1	Severe Problem	Poor understanding; not open to educational intervention.
0	Not Assessed	Subject has no family or social worker is unable (or it is inappropriate) to rate family understanding at the time of assessment.

Source: Reprinted with permission from RIC-FAS V, p. 72, Copyright © 1987, 1989, 1992, 1996, 1998.

social worker family interview as well as information gained by other team members will often identify these needs. Additionally, a self-administered assessment instrument, such as the Family Needs Questionnaire that can be filled out in a private, quiet, and reflective moment can add depth to the team's knowledge of what the family members feel they need.[7] The Family Needs Questionnaire was designed for families of individuals suffering from traumatic brain injury; however, most of its questions are applicable to other diagnoses as well. It consists of 40 self-administered questions that ask the family member to indicate how important it is to have a particular need met by circling a number on a 1

Exhibit 6–4 Family Adaptation Scale

Includes family's adjustment to disability including coping, stage of family life cycle, effective and consistent communication, flexibility of family roles, tolerance of individuality, self-esteem, and relationship to counseling interventions.

Scale Points	Level	Behavioral Definition
7	No Problem	No counseling needs identified.
6	Minimal Problem	Coping well, but could benefit from supportive contacts.
5	Mild Problem	Some difficulty coping; would benefit from counseling intervention.
4	Mild to Moderate Problem	Coping difficulties on a daily basis, complicated by chronic dysfunction or other stressors.
3	Moderate Problem	Poor coping; may complicate rehabilitation and discharge planning; limits family involvement.
2	Moderate to Severe Problem	Coping interferes with rehabilitation and planning; precludes family involvement.
1	Severe Problem	Extreme difficulty coping; psychiatric intervention/hospitalization needed on an emergency basis (may be related to premorbid difficulties).
0	Not Assessed	Subject has no family or social worker is unable (or it is inappropriate) to rate family adaptation at the time of assessment.

Source: Reprinted with permission from RIC-FAS V, p. 73, Copyright © 1987, 1989, 1992, 1996, 1998.

to 5 scale with 5 being very important. The individual can also indicate whether the need has been met, partially met, or not met and can also indicate those needs that are not applicable. The questions focus on the following six areas of potential need:

1. Need for medical information. (Example: "I need to have complete information on the medical care of the client," or "I need to know how long each of the client's problems is expected to last.")

Exhibit 6–5 Support Network Scale

Includes the amount of support and availability of the subject's family/ support network. Measures the degree of, or problems with, support and availability.

Scale Points	Level	Behavioral Definition
7	No Problem	Family/significant individuals are supportive and available with no identified problems. (Consistently provide support and accept responsibility for follow-through of care needs.)
6	Minimal Problem	Family/significant individuals are supportive and available, but are dealing with competing commitments that limit involvement with subject.
5	Mild Problem	Family/significant individuals are supportive but have limited availability (due to geographic distance and other family problems).
4	Mild to Moderate Problem	Family/significant individuals have difficulty providing support to subject due to reactions to disability issues.
3	Moderate Problem	Family/significant individuals are minimally involved. Family/significant individuals have difficulty providing support due to preexisting dysfunction.
2	Moderate to Severe Problem	Family/significant individuals are rarely involved, unable or unwilling to provide support.
1	Severe Problem	Subject has no identified support network.
0	Not Assessed	Social worker is unable (or it is inappropriate) to rate support network at the time of the assessment.

Source: Reprinted with permission from RIC-FAS V, p. 25, Copyright © 1987, 1989, 1992, 1996, 1998.

2. Need for emotional support. (Example: "I need to know if I am making the best possible decisions about the patient," or "I need to have my spouse understand how difficult it is for me.")
3. Need for instrumental support (e.g., housekeeping, shopping, child care, transportation help). (Example: "I need help keeping the house," or "I need to have enough resources for myself or the family [e.g., financial or legal counseling, respite care, counseling, nursing, or day care].)
4. Need for professional support. (Example: "I need to have a professional to turn to for advice or services when the patient needs help," or "I need to have different staff members agree on the best way to help the patient.")
5. Need for patient support. (Example: "I need to be assured that the best possible medical care is being provided," or "I need to be shown that medical, educational, or rehabilitation staff respect the client's needs or wishes.")
6. Need for involvement with client care. (Example: "I need to be told daily what is being done for the client," or "I need to give my opinions daily to others involved in the client's care or rehabilitation.")

Identify Required Logistical Supports

Each family will need some logistical support in order to successfully maintain the client's achieved outcome after discharge. The type and amount of support that families will need in order to plan for and procure community resources will vary. The types of supports should be identified as early as possible in the rehabilitation process so the family can make connections with the source of support well in advance of the client's discharge. Some of the more common areas of needed logistical support are:

- Health care
  1. Medical support—Identify and clarify health care access criteria, guidelines, and processes required by the client's health care plan. Identify the physician within the health care plan that will follow the client after discharge. Identify when and how to make physician appointments. Identify how to question coverage decisions made by the health care plan.

2. General health—Identify appropriate wellness programs that can help with prevention of identified risk factors.
3. Residential support—Identify home modifications, equipment, and supplies that will be required and the vendors for each. Link up family with vendors. Ensure that the family knows how to obtain any residential supports that will be needed on an ongoing basis. Ensure that the family is aware of appropriate residential options (including names, addresses, and phone numbers) in the event that after discharge they find they cannot adequately support the client at home.

- Family support—Identify family/client support systems such as immediate and extended family, friends, and resources through their religious and/or organizational affiliations. Prior to discharge, facilitate a linkage and support plan with the support system the family has identified that is appropriate for them. Identify leisure resources that are appropriate to the family's or client's past or present interests and ability to access them; facilitate family linkage with them prior to discharge. Where appropriate, identify respite resources, access requirements, and family linkage with them.
- Community support—Identify and create family linkage with appropriate support groups, crisis counseling, in-home services, low- or no-cost continued therapy services where indicated, and transportation services to assist in accessing community resources.
- Financial support—Identify financial resources that may be available within the client's health care plan to support either partially or fully any of the required supports identified above, ways to access them, and any restrictions or required copayments. Identify any local, state, and/ or federal financial resources for which the client or the family qualifies and facilitate the linkage with these resources.

Family Management Plan Development

As stated earlier, the goal of the family management plan is to avoid client regression after discharge due to the development of a codependency between the client and family members. In order to reach this primary goal, the team must meet the following objectives:

- facilitate active involvement of the client's family in the rehabilitation process
- facilitate family understanding of and adaptation to the effects of the client's disabilities on the family system
- provide the family with the emotional and practical tools required to sustain the client's outcome after discharge

To meet these objectives, the rehabilitation team develops the family rehabilitation plan around the following three components:

1. *The disabilities that must be treated.* These include the family needs that must be met and the family supports that will be required. The information derived from the Family Needs Questionnaire and identified logistical support that the family requires defines the family disabilities that must be treated.

2. *The type and amount of intervention required to meet the family needs and provide the required supports.* The type and amount of counseling, education, and training is based on the family's understanding of and adjustment to disability and the strength of its support network. The information obtained from the Family Understanding of Disability Scale, the Family Adaptation Scale, and the Family Assessment Device identifies the type and amount of intervention that is appropriate for meeting the needs of each family member and the different needs of each family.

3. *The timing of the interventions.* The timing of interventions is based on the family's emotional status at any given point in time. The family's emotional status directly affects its ability to receive, understand, integrate, learn, and perform approaches and techniques that will assist in the rehabilitation process and support the attained outcome after discharge. The information derived from the identification of the family members' phases of response to disablement and their stage of grieving will provide guideposts as to when it is best to provide certain types of education, skills training, and counseling.

CLARIFY ROLES AND EXPECTATIONS

The team implements the family rehabilitation plan within the context of three therapeutic procedures: (1) it must simultaneously facilitate an

atmosphere of a partnership with the family, (2) provide the right education and training at appropriate times, and (3) ensure that all interactions
with the family are therapeutic in nature.

Historically, the team has viewed the family as passive recipients of its
knowledge and expertise. For a typical family, the greatest degree of
involvement in the rehabilitation process is learning how to support a
client's home exercise program. To do this, therapists provided verbal
instruction, visual demonstrations, and written instructions that are often
combined with pictures. Having provided this information, the family
practices the techniques until they can successfully "reverse demonstrate"
them to the therapist. Certainly, the family's ability to supervise and
support the home exercise program is an important aspect of its involvement in the rehabilitation process. This goal, however, falls far short of
providing the family with all the emotional, educational, and practical
tools it will need to participate successfully in a client's rehabilitation
program and support the outcome after discharge. The family must become true partners with the team in the rehabilitation process. They must
be facilitated to become active decision-making partners—partners in
deciding what, when, and how services are delivered both to the client and
themselves. To achieve an atmosphere of partnership, the team must
facilitate within the family a sense of internal locus of control and maintain
open channels of communication.

Facilitate Internal Locus of Control

Most families have no prior experience with rehabilitation. As a consequence, they typically respond to it in a manner similar to their previous
health care experiences. In their previous experience, they have gone to a
physician who diagnosed their problem and performed the medical intervention necessary to alleviate it. They were the passive recipients of a
"cure" for their medical problem. When they find themselves confronted
with a medical problem that requires rehabilitation, they behave in the only
way they know how—they turn the responsibility for recovery over to the
physicians and therapists. They expect the complete recovery that has
resulted from their previous health care experiences and expect to be
passive participants in the process. Families often hold expectations such
as:

- Rehabilitation will make my family member just as he or she was before.
- I turn my family member over to you, the experts, to cure.
- Rehabilitation will free me from having to take care of my family member.
- If my family member is not in treatment all the time, he or she will not get better.
- Only individual therapy will help.
- Treatment should continue as long as he or she has impairments.
- Therapy must be provided only by the therapist (the expert), not an aide.
- The professional should provide the amount and duration of therapy the client needs regardless of what my health care policy will pay for.

Discuss Expectations

Such expectations are all symptomatic of the family's sense of external locus of control—that is, the belief that therapists and physicians will meet the client's needs and that they have no personal responsibility for, nor influence on, the outcome of the services that are provided. To successfully achieve a sense of partnership with the family, the team members must facilitate a sense of internal locus of control between the family and the team.[8] The team must help the family believe that it can and must influence the outcome, both for its sake and the client's. Internal locus of control can be facilitated by clarifying the expectations of all parties, clarifying rights and responsibilities, recognizing, respecting, and utilizing the family's expertise, and ensuring that the family understands the day-to-day process and logistics of rehabilitation.

All parties involved in the rehabilitation process hold expectations of what the outcome will be and what each other's roles will be in achieving that outcome. It is essential to discuss openly and—where indicated—refine or redefine the expectations each party holds for themselves and the others. At minimum, the following expectations should be discussed and clarified with the family:

- the team's perception of the expected client outcome and the family's perception of the expected outcome

- what the team is able to do to help the client reach the expected outcome and what the family expects the team to do
- what the team expects the family to do to help the client attain and sustain the expected outcome
- what the team expects the client to do to attain and maintain the expected outcome and what the family expects the client to do
- the amount of postdischarge ongoing caregiver support the team expects the family to provide and what the family expects to provide

The clarification of these expectations is absolutely essential to the facilitation of the family's understanding and acceptance of the reality that rehabilitation does not "cure" impairments and their attendant disabilities. This process helps impart the knowledge that, with family assistance, improvement can continue after discharge from therapy. It creates an understanding that a point will be reached in the rehabilitation process when "skilled therapy" will no longer be required for the client to continue improving. The process of clarifying expectations also begins to help the family to understand and emotionally deal with the fact that a point will be reached where continued intervention will no longer benefit the client and that the client will always have some degree of chronic disability. The acknowledgment and acceptance of those facts are critical to the family's ability to realistically plan for the client's discharge from rehabilitation and will determine the family's readiness to learn the skills it will need to provide the client with appropriate help and avoid over- or underhelping after discharge.

Recognize, Respect, and Utilize the Family's Expertise

The family holds a wealth of invaluable information that the team can use to understand the client's reaction to and manner of participation in rehabilitation. The family knows the client's personal preferences regarding basic things such as food, beverages, temperature, sleep needs, and sleep patterns. It knows the client's attitude toward and reaction to illness as well as toward pain and frustration tolerance. It can tell the team about the client's degree of need for privacy and whether he or she was a person who enjoyed interacting with people or preferred solo activities. The family can give the team insight to the client's goals, aspirations, and values as well as sources of internal and external motivation and strength.

The family is the expert about the person who is the team's client. The family can train the team on how best to approach and work with the client.

Explain the Process and Logistics of Rehabilitation

The family is in foreign territory and often confused by all that is going on around them. To participate in the rehabilitation process, the family must have an understanding of how it works. For example, family members need to understand the whys and hows of the therapy scheduling process, the assignment of therapists to cases, and changes in therapists. They need to know when, why, and how assistants/aides will be used, as well as why cotreatment and group therapy may be used in conjunction with or in place of individual therapy. They need to know why personal care is scheduled by nursing at certain times and not others. They need to understand the role of the physician in relationship to the role of the therapists.

CLARIFY CLIENT RIGHTS AND RESPONSIBILITIES

Because of the nature of many rehabilitation conditions, clients are not always able to independently understand and/or monitor staff compliance with their rights, nor are they able to independently understand and/or comply with their responsibilities. As a consequence, families are often the client's surrogate with respect to monitoring compliance with rights and responsibilities. Because of this, the team should proactively encourage the family to immediately discuss with the designated staff member any concerns regarding staff compliance with their family members' rights and to also immediately discuss client compliance concerns both with the client and the team. Exhibit 6–6 provides an example of a statement of such rights and responsibilities.

MAINTAIN OPEN COMMUNICATION

The first step in open communication is the use of terminology that the family can understand. Common everyday terms and descriptions should replace professional jargon. When a professional term must be used, it

Exhibit 6–6 Client Rights and Responsibilities

Rights
1. You have the right to considerate, professional, and respectful care, regardless of age, sex, race, color, religion, national origin, nature of illness, or source of payment.
2. You have the right to know who is attending to you and why someone is performing a particular task. You may question all persons involved with your care regarding their function or the purpose of the service they provide.
3. You have the right to expect reasonable continuity of care.
4. You have the right to expect the hospital to make a reasonable response to your requests.
5. You have the right to obtain information from your physician regarding the appropriateness of your admission.
6. You have the right to receive from your physician and therapists complete and current information concerning your diagnosis, treatment, and prognosis in terms you can reasonably be expected to understand.
7. You have the right to receive from your physician and therapists information necessary to give informed consent prior to the start of any procedure and/or treatment.
8. You have the right to every consideration of your privacy concerning your own medical care program.
9. You have the right to choose not to have visitors.
10. You have the right to refuse treatment to the extent permitted by law, and to be informed of the consequences of your actions.
11. You have the right to be provided information by your physician regarding educational, experimental, and research projects related to your case; you may refuse to participate in any of these projects.
12. You have the right to expect that all communications and records pertaining to your care should be treated as confidential. You may review or obtain a copy of your medical record by contacting the Medical Records Department.
13. You have the right to obtain information as to any relationship of the hospital to other health care and educational institutions insofar as your care is concerned.
14. You have the right to be informed of any rules or regulations of the hospital that apply to your conduct as a patient.
15. You have the right to examine and receive an explanation of your bill, regardless of the source of payment.

continues

Exhibit 6–6 continued

Responsibilities

1. You have the responsibility to provide, to the best of your knowledge, accurate and complete information about present complaints, past illnesses, medications, hospitalizations, and other matters relating to your health, and to report unexpected changes in your condition to those involved in your care.

2. You have the responsibility to cooperate with all hospital staff caring for you, and to ask questions if you do not understand directions or instructions given to you.

3. You have the responsibility to help the hospital staff in their efforts to help you by following their instructions and medical orders.

4. You have the responsibility to follow and maintain the treatment recommended by your physician and therapists after you are discharged from the hospital.

5. You and your visitors have the responsibility to abide by the hospital rules and regulations, and to be respectful and considerate of other persons, other persons' property, and the property of the hospital. You and your visitors should be especially aware of the hospital rules regarding smoking.

6. You have the responsibility to keep appointments and to contact the appropriate member of the staff within a reasonable amount of time if you cannot keep an appointment.

7. You have the responsibility to contact the appropriate staff member as quickly as possible if you believe that any of these rights or responsibilities have not or cannot be fulfilled.

8. You have the responsibility to be timely in your payment of hospital bills, to provide the information necessary for insurance billing, and to ask questions concerning the bill as soon as possible.

---

should be accompanied by a definition and a determination whether or not the family understood the definition within the context of the client's rehabilitation goals. Next, it is extremely important that the family knows how to obtain the information it needs and whom to seek out for decisions. It is often helpful to designate one member of the team as the family liaison. The liaison can serve the family by communicating with and/or obtaining answers from various team members.

Family expectations will change across the course of rehabilitation in relation to the speed and degree of improvement observed. As a result of what the family observes and learns from the team, it may raise or lower its expectations. In some instances, families who originally thought they would be able to take the client home, begin to feel that they won't be able to. The opposite also occurs when families decide they will be capable of supporting the client at home, when at first they thought they could not. Because expectations change, it is of paramount importance that the team proactively continue the process of clarifying expectations during the course of rehabilitation. Finally, the team should conduct periodic customer satisfaction surveys during the course of rehabilitation. Not all families feel comfortable discussing sources of dissatisfaction while they are still involved in the rehabilitation program. By proactively asking for satisfaction feedback during rehabilitation, the team not only keeps the door to communication open but creates the opportunity to remedy client care problems while they are occurring rather than hearing about them after discharge. At minimum, the customer satisfaction survey should cover the areas of satisfaction with the rehabilitation process, education and training, and hospitality. Exhibit 6–7 includes sample questions that the rehabilitation team could ask families regarding the three areas cited above.

PROVIDE EDUCATION AND TRAINING

The client's ability to maintain or enhance the rehabilitation outcome after discharge depends heavily upon the family's ability to provide the required caregiving, therapy maintenance, and support in an appropriate manner and amount, and at the appropriate time. The education and training approach that the team utilizes, as well as the timing of when they offer it, is critical to the family's ability to learn when and how to provide assistance. Under the best of circumstances, learning something that is completely foreign takes time. Under stressful conditions, learning will be slow and erratic. Information is often retained in disjointed fragments that are partially composed of what was taught, partially of what the individual believed he or she was told or saw, and partially the way the individual personally believes things should be done. The degree of inaccuracy, misperception, and misrepresentation will be proportional to the degree of stress the family is under at any given time.

Exhibit 6–7 Sample Questions for Customer Satisfaction Survey

Satisfaction with the rehabilitation process:
- Do you feel you have been sufficiently informed about your family member's condition and progress?
- Do you feel you are being sufficiently involved in decisions regarding your family member's rehabilitation goals and program?
- Do you feel your suggestions are respected and utilized in your family member's rehabilitation program?
- Does the progress made so far by your family member meet your expectations?

Satisfaction with education and training:
- Does the education and training you are receiving make sense to you?
- Do you feel that the education and training is providing you with the skills you need?
- Are your questions being answered clearly and completely?
- Are you feeling confident and competent to perform the skills you are being taught?
- Are the written materials and illustrations provided to you helpful?

Hospitality:
- Do you feel you are being treated with respect?
- Are your concerns or complaints being handled courteously?
- Are your concerns or complaints being handled effectively?
- Is the environment clean and comfortable for you?

Educating and Training at the Right Time

Consequently, the family must be emotionally ready to receive the information it needs to participate in learning the techniques that must be employed. If they are not emotionally ready, they will not be in a position to mentally engage themselves in the instructions they receive. If they are not mentally ready to engage in the learning process, they will not be able to internalize the information and techniques presented by the therapist, and, consequently, will not be able to retrieve and use the information at a later date. Therapists cannot assume that learning has taken place simply because they provided information, instructions, and/or demonstrations of the caregiving and maintenance techniques that the client will need after discharge. It is entirely possible for a family member to "reverse demon-strate" a technique or to repeat information to a therapist and not to have actually learned the techniques and information.

Educating and Training in the Right Way

Quite frequently counseling is the first step toward successful family education and training and most often must continue parallel to it. Assist-ing the family with the grieving process, as well as their understanding of and adaptation to disability, lays the groundwork for the family to attend to, learn, and use the information and skills training they need. For example, families that are in the shock or denial stage of grieving are in no emotional position to engage in education and training. Similarly, family members who are at Level 4 or below on the Family Understanding of Disability Scale (Exhibit 6–3) or Level 3 or below on the Family Adapta-tion Scale (Exhibit 6–4) also are not yet in a position to learn. Not all family members are in the same stage of grieving or at the same level of understanding of and adaptation to disability at the same time. As a consequence, the social worker or psychologist must quickly identify a member of the family who is ready for learning so that education and training can commence as early as possible in the rehabilitation process.

Knowledge and skills are best learned in the context of actual experi-ence. Education and training should be provided within the context of the client's treatment sessions. During the treatment session, the therapist can explain the rationale behind each technique, demonstrate it, and discuss it with the family. When the family indicates that it understands the rationale and purpose of the techniques, the therapist can take them through the procedures in a hand-over-hand manner. This learning process is repeated until family members not only demonstrate their proficiency in providing the techniques, but also report that they feel confident and competent to do so on their own. A multisystems teaching approach should be used to assist the family in the learning process. Besides education and training, the family should receive written and graphic instructional material and how-to instructional videos or audiotapes. If possible, family members should have the opportunity to talk to families who have already gone through the process. Peer coaching is a very powerful teaching tool. Peer coaches can provide variations on techniques that they have found fit the unique and, sometimes, unforeseen demands of their real-world environment.

Not all individuals learn in the same manner. Some learn best through verbal instruction, some through visual demonstrations; others learn only by doing, and still others may require combinations of all three modes of learning. An individual's mode of learning also may be different for different types of information. It is the therapist's responsibility to identify and utilize each family member's unique style of learning. As the client progresses through the various phases of rehabilitation, therapists must also be prepared to answer the same questions over and over and to repeat the same skill training until the family finally understands the process and has mastered and performed the required skills with ease. The fact that family members have difficulty retaining and applying what they have learned does not mean that they are difficult, uncooperative, or unmotivated. Most frequently it means that they are having difficulty coping with the drastic changes that have occurred in their lives. It is in this context that the therapist can apply the knowledge gained through identifying family members' needs, their level of understanding of the client's condition, their level of adjustment to it, and their existing support network.

Facilitating a Therapeutic Relationship

The key to successful family rehabilitation is not the education and training provided per se but rather the quality of the interactions that occur between the therapist and the family. Every interaction is a family rehabilitation opportunity. Success is more often found in how the therapist interacts with the family than in what the interaction is about. A family's willingness and ability to participate in the treatment plan depends heavily upon the therapist's ability to facilitate a therapeutic relationship—one in which the family feels absolutely comfortable in questioning, challenging, and disagreeing with the therapist, therapy techniques, or the condition and progress of their family member. Such a relationship can evolve only when the therapist understands that all such interactions are not personal challenges but rather expressions of the family's hopes and fears. They are expressions that take on the tone of the family members' stages of grieving as well as their understanding of and adjustment to their family member's disabilities. Such interactions not only are opportunities to respond to and meet family needs but are also opportunities to assist the family with its grieving and adjustment to the disabilities of the family member. To facilitate a therapeutic relationship, the therapist needs both an understanding of how the family may enter the relationship, as well as the ability to respond to questions, challenges, and disagreements in a therapeutic manner.

Most relationships are entered into out of individual choice. This, however, is not the case in the relationship between therapist and family. Neither party chose to be in a relationship. The consequences of a medical condition has brought them together as a *fait accompli*. The family did not want the medical episode and the therapist did not request to treat the client. Both parties have different starting points in their relationship with the client as well as different types of emotional investment in that relationship. The family has a long history with the client and the therapist's relationship with the client begins upon admission to rehabilitation. The family is attached to and emotionally involved with its family member and the therapist is emotionally invested in helping the client to improve as well as in providing the services that the therapist has been trained to provide. As a consequence, the family can become easily offended if the therapist's manner of relating is viewed as inconsistent with the needs, wants, sensitivities, and abilities of the person they have known for so long. Given this starting point in the relationship, it is important that therapists are sensitive to the fact that, even though the client is in their rehabilitation facility, they are, from the family's perspective, entering into the family's territory. Knowing this, the therapist should solicit the family's recommendations as how best to approach and interact with the client. If the client has been at another level of care, the therapist should obtain from family members their knowledge about the previous care and do things that way, if appropriate in relation to the client's current status, or inform them how and why things will be different. The therapist should always prepare the family in advance for changes in routines and procedures, especially procedures that may cause pain, discomfort, frustration, or anger.

One of the most frequently cited family needs is the desire for information.[9,10] The family responses to the Family Needs Questionnaire (discussed earlier in this chapter) can provide the team with specific areas of needed information. Once identified, the information should be provided immediately to the family. The information should be shared privately and with sensitivity and care. Regular family-team meetings are an essential mode of sharing information. These meetings provide family members with continual progress updates, a chance to hear from all disciplines at once, and a chance to have their questions and concerns addressed as well as to participate in the planning process. Finally, because discharge from rehabilitation can be a very stressful time for the family, it is critical for the team to discuss the projected discharge date, place of discharge, and postdischarge plans at frequent intervals throughout rehabilitation. A difficult concept for the family to grasp and accept is that of "medical necessity." This concept, which was presented Chapter 5, must be explained to the family early in the rehabilitation process and discussed at all following family conferences. A family's lack of understanding or acceptance of the fact that continued rehabilitation must be based on medical necessity is one of the more frequent sources of conflict between therapists and families.

Resolving Conflicts

The manner in which the therapist handles questions, challenges, demands, and disagreements is critical to the development and maintenance of a therapeutic therapist/family relationship. If the therapist interprets the family's behavior as a personal challenge to the therapist's competence, then the interaction will take on a defensive tone and a sense within the family that the therapist is more concerned about his or her ego than about meeting their needs. On the other hand, if the therapist interprets family behavior as a source of guidance, the therapist will be able to meet the family's needs. The following is one method of dealing with a distraught family member:[11]

1. *Find the best environment to talk.* Find a place where the family member will feel comfortable to talk freely. Do not talk in a hallway, around other people, or in closed spaces or rooms stored with a lot of medical equipment. Also, find a place where you will not be interrupted. Do not sit behind a desk or table, as that is perceived as distancing.

2. *Listen.* Do not give explanations or make excuses. Listen and identify the problem. Problems usually involve one of the following areas: the care of the client, perception of staff's ability or level of caring, client condition or prognosis, relationship issues with staff or other family members, and finances. Frequently the problem that is stated is not the real problem. The real problem may very well relate to the family member's stage of grieving or understanding of and adjustment to their family member's disability. Regardless, the stated problem must be addressed first.

3. *Reassure*. Reassurance comes in part from dealing with the stated problem, but also through answering questions and providing information.

4. *Develop an action plan*. Strategize together. To facilitate this process, ask questions such as, "What would you like to see happen?" or "What would make it better?" You may not be the person to solve the problem. Do not promise anything beyond your authority. If the solution lies with someone outside your authority, plan to arrange a meeting with the person who has the authority to solve the problem.

5. *Follow up*. Thank the family member for bringing up the problem and give your assurances that you are always available to listen to and try to solve problems. Identify a backup resource person for when you might be unavailable. Continue to follow up on the action plan. Find the family member on visits or by phone and communicate the results of the action plan and solicit the family member's perception about whether the problem has been resolved. Go back to step one again if the plan was not effective.

6. During the course of resolving the stated problem, the family member may bring forward information that suggests that there is a deeper problem. If this occurs, the family member should be encouraged to discuss it with the social worker or psychologist.

Successful conflict resolution calls upon the therapist to understand that the existence of a conflict is a therapeutic opportunity rather than a personal affront or attack. It is the therapist's responsibility to his or her client to first create a therapeutic atmosphere and then to take a leadership role in resolving the conflict. A therapeutic atmosphere arises when the therapist functions from the premise that the family member is right from his or her perspective. The leadership role is that of respecting the family member's perspective and working to find a solution to the problem that meets the needs of all involved. To achieve such a solution, the therapist must approach his or her therapeutic conflict resolution responsibility from the perspective that when a difference exists between two parties, there is no right or wrong, good or bad point of view. Instead, each point of view is both right and wrong and good and bad. Each position taken will be right and good for some who are involved in the conflict and that which is right and good for them may very well be wrong and bad for the other parties who are involved. The therapy goal in conflict resolution is to find a win-win resolution for all parties.

CONCLUSION

The previous two chapters have focused on the client management components of the MORsystem. This chapter addressed what, in many respects, is the most important component of the MORsystem: the management of the family's needs throughout the rehabilitation process. The client is a member of a cohesive family unit, a unit that becomes disrupted in the face of a catastrophic medical episode. In the final analysis, after the intervention of the rehabilitation professionals has been completed, it is the family that will be called upon to reinforce the outcome that has been achieved. The family members will be responsible for facilitating the client's reintegration into the family unit and, ultimately, into the community. Most certainly, then, it is the family that plays the pivotal role in the ultimate success or failure of all of the rehabilitation efforts that have converged to produce the client's outcome. It is the family that will determine the durability and value of the outcome that has been achieved. In this context, the family is the vital link to the rehabilitation team's ability to produce an outcome with the highest cost/benefit ratio. It is imperative, then, that the team understand that it cannot treat successfully the client without simultaneously treating the family unit as well. The team must direct its efforts toward the impact of the medical episode on the entire family in order to minimize the risk of client/family codependency after discharge from rehabilitation. In other words, the achieved outcome most predictably will deteriorate if, after discharge, the client obtains help from the family that is not needed in relation to his or her regained abilities or if the family provides unsolicited and unneeded assistance. To avoid codependency, the team must establish a family management plan in parallel with the client's management plan. The purpose and goal of the family management plan is to facilitate a sense of internal locus of control within all members of the family.

REFERENCES

1. R. McNeny and P. Wilcox, Partners by Force: The Family and the Rehabilitation Team, *NeuroRehabilitation 1*, no. 2 (1991): 7–17.
2. E. Kubler-Ross, *On Death and Dying* (New York: Macmillan Publishing USA, 1969), 38–138.
3. Rehabilitation Institute of Chicago, *Functional Assessment Scale Version IV* (Chicago: 1996), 73.

4. Rehabilitation Institute of Chicago, *Functional Assessment Scale*, 72.

5. Rehabilitation Institute of Chicago, *Functional Assessment Scale*, 25.

6. N. Epstein et al., The McMaster Family Assessment Device, *Journal of Marital and Family Therapy 9*, no. 2 (1983): 171–180.

7. A. Witol et al., A Longitudinal Analysis of Family Needs following Traumatic Brain Injury, *NeuroRehabilitation 7* (1996): 175–187.

8. G. Fawcett et al., Locus of Control, Perceived Constraint, and Morale among Institutionalized Aged, *International Journal on Aging and Human Development 11*, no. 1 (1980).

9. J. Bluhm, Helping Families in Crisis Hold On, *Nursing 17* (1987): 44–48.

10. L. Shaw and McMahon, Family–Staff Conflict in the Rehabilitation Setting: Causes, Consequences, and Implications, *Brain Injury 4* (1990): 87–93.

11. C. Elizabeth, Coping with the Difficult Family Member: A Model, *Family Relations* (December 1987): 32–33.

CHAPTER 7

Team Management Tools

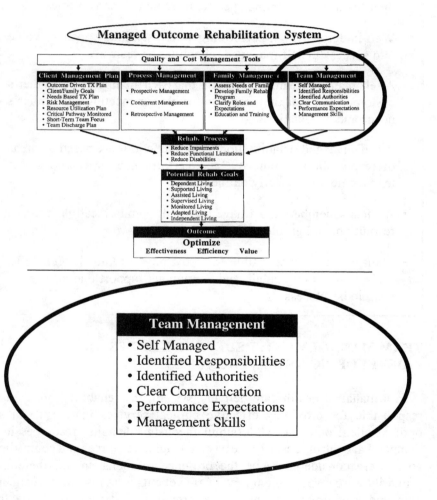

Managed Outcome Rehabilitation System

Quality and Cost Management Tools

Client Management Plan
- Outcome Driven TX Plan
- Client/Family Goals
- Needs Based TX Plan
- Risk Management
- Resource Utilization Plan
- Critical Pathway Monitored
- Short-Term Team Focus
- Team Discharge Plan

Process Management
- Prospective Management
- Concurrent Management
- Retrospective Management

Family Management
- Assess Needs of Family
- Develop Family Rehab Program
- Clarify Roles and Expectations
- Education and Training

Team Management
- Self Managed
- Identified Responsibilities
- Identified Authorities
- Clear Communication
- Performance Expectations
- Management Skills

Rehab. Process
- Reduce Impairments
- Reduce Functional Limitations
- Reduce Disabilities

Potential Rehab Goals
- Dependent Living
- Supported Living
- Assisted Living
- Supervised Living
- Monitored Living
- Adapted Living
- Independent Living

Outcome
Optimize
Effectiveness   Efficiency   Value

Team Management
- Self Managed
- Identified Responsibilities
- Identified Authorities
- Clear Communication
- Performance Expectations
- Management Skills

KEY POINTS:

- Effective and efficient management of the rehabilitation process requires a self-managed team that is empowered by management to make timely clinical, financial, and personnel decisions.

- For a team to become self-managed, its members must relinquish their historical discipline-specific roles and responsibilities.

- Well-integrated high-performing interdisciplinary teams evolve into successful self-managed rehabilitation teams.

- A self-managed team understands that each member is each other's customer and that they are responsible for meeting each other's needs and expectations.

- A self-managed rehabilitation team's functions are based on areas of responsibility, authority, and performance expectations that management has clearly defined.

- All team members must have excellent communication, conflict resolution, and problem-solving skills.

- Management is responsible for providing the knowledge, skills, tools, work environment, and continuous support that allows the team to be successful.

TEAM MANAGEMENT: REDEFINING ROLES AND DEVELOPING NEW APPROACHES

In a managed health care delivery system, the rehabilitation team is responsible for providing effective clinical services that result in an optimal client outcome while simultaneously managing resources in a manner that controls costs. In the past, managing resources and controlling costs were considered to be the province of management; therapists primarily were responsible for evaluating clients, establishing a treatment plan, and providing treatment that was effective. Under managed care, the cost control responsibility has shifted from management to the therapists as individuals and to the team as a whole. Clinical decisions now are also financial decisions. For this reason, the team must organize and control the provision of its services to achieve client-specific outcomes within fiscally responsible time frames while using only those resources that are absolutely necessary to achieve the expected outcome. To meet their responsibilities successfully, all team members must continually communicate, collaborate, coordinate, and problem solve. The Managed Outcome Rehabilitation System (MORsystem) provides the framework, process, and tools required to make service quality and cost decisions at the team level. The intricacy and immediacy of communication, collaboration, coordination, and problem solving that will be required, however, necessitates that the team be capable of collective self-management. Therapists are used to managing themselves within the boundaries of the roles and responsibilities of their respective disciplines. At the team level of service delivery, however, therapists are used to depending upon an appointed leader, both within the team and within specialty departments, to address and handle issues of interdisciplinary service coordination, productivity, and costs. These "management" responsibilities now become team responsibilities—the rehabilitation team must now manage itself. This does not mean the absence of a leader, but rather a change in the roles and expectations of the team leader and team members. As shown in Figure 7–1, the role of the team leader is now significantly different. The team leader is a:

- Leader: one who leads by empowering the team to be the primary decision makers by facilitating them to create a team vision, goals, objectives, and expected results both at the client, team, and program level
- Coach: one who teaches others and helps them develop their potential; maintains a balance of authority among the team members, and ensures the accountability of all team members to each other, the client, employer, and payer
- Business analyzer: one who understands the big picture and is able to translate changes in the greater business environment into opportunities for the organization as a whole
- Barrier buster: one who opens doors and runs interference for the team and breaks down artificial barriers in order for the team to be successful
- Facilitator: one who brings together the necessary tools, information, and resources for the team to get the job done and facilitates group efforts

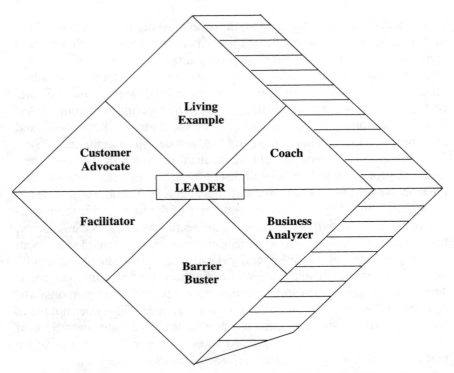

Figure 7–1 Team Leader Role. *Source:* Copyright © Belgard • Fisher • Rayner, Inc.

- Customer advocate: one who develops and maintains close customer (client, employer, and payer) ties, articulates customer needs, and keeps priorities in focus with the desires and expectations of the customer
- Living example: one who serves as a role model for others by "walking the walk," demonstrates the desired behaviors of team members and leaders[1]

Just as the roles and expectations of the leader of a self-managed rehabilitation team are significantly different, so too are the roles and responsibilities of team members. As shown in Figure 7–2, each member of the team is a:

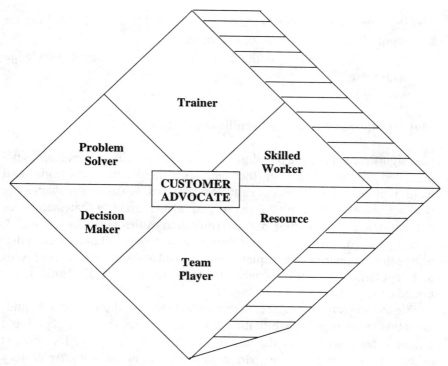

Figure 7–2 Team Member Role. *Source:* Copyright © Belgard • Fisher • Rayner, Inc.

- Customer advocate: constantly and continually strives to better meet the needs of the customer
- Skilled worker: demonstrates all the necessary skills and knowledge to perform the specialty job well; continually strives to improve specialty skills to ensure quality of service
- Resource: has a diverse and ever-expanding set of skills; continually broadens knowledge base in order to bring more than expected specialty skills to bear on a client's rehabilitation
- Team player: demonstrates good interpersonal skills; supports other team members
- Decision maker: provides input and makes decisions on issues that directly affect and enhance the work of all team members

- Problem solver: understands and utilizes problem-solving techniques regularly to identify and solve problems
- Trainer: trains others on the team and continually shares knowledge with them[2]

Multidisciplinary vs. Interdisciplinary Teams

A significant change, a paradigm shift, will be required to develop a self-managed rehabilitation team that embodies these new team leader and team member roles, functions, and expectations. A paradigm shapes the way we see the world. It is a sort of map of the territory that shapes our perceptions, understanding, and interpretation of the world around us.[3] A paradigm, then, is a set of societal, community, group, or family values that define the boundaries of acceptable actions and activities and a set of rules and regulations that tell us what to do to be successful within those boundaries.

The fee-for-service health care reimbursement paradigm created boundaries that encouraged rehabilitation teams to produce the highest possible outcome no matter what the cost. Consequently, the rules for success within the boundaries of this paradigm are found in the *multidisciplinary* team approach to rehabilitation. In this approach, the client is viewed as a constellation of separate impairments that are treated within the boundaries of the historically rigid roles and functions of each discipline on the team. The *multidisciplinary* team approach fosters the development of discipline-specific long- and short-term goals but not the treatment toward a unifying non–discipline-specific whole person goal. It also relies on the team leader to make decisions regarding the medical necessity of each discipline's service as well as to identify and problem solve gaps that occur between services and across levels of care. The multidisciplinary team approach will not produce successful teams within the boundaries of the managed care paradigm. The multidisciplinary team approach creates an atmosphere of territoriality, turf, fragmentation of the client's needs, and a "that's not my job" attitude, which are ineffective and inefficient.

The boundaries and values of the managed care paradigm also demand the attainment of the highest possible outcome, but at the least cost. Quality service based on controlled costs that results in optimal outcomes can only be realized through a self-managed *interdisciplinary* team service delivery paradigm. Successful teams within a managed care environment will be those who function as a well-integrated interdisciplinary team. Such teams view the client as a whole person with disabilities that cross discipline boundaries. An *interdisciplinary* team has flexible definitions of roles and functions that allow for the overlapping of services, which, in turn, facilitates continuity of care across disciplines. Ultimately, the interdisciplinary team must evolve into a high-performing self-managed interdisciplinary team. A team in which all members are accountable for the client's attainment of the expected whole person outcome, within the expected length of stay, and at or below the expected cost. To respond to this accountability, high-performing teams rely upon self-directed group collaboration and self-directed and proactive problem solving. Today, high-performing interdisciplinary teamwork is a business necessity and a job requirement.

THE SELF-MANAGED REHABILITATION TEAM (SMRT): MAKING THE PARADIGM SHIFT

Shifting from a multidisciplinary team approach to a self-managed interdisciplinary team approach is like being traded from a baseball team to a football team: Each sport has its own unique rules and regulations and measurements for success. If you analyze each type of team on the variables of autonomy, initiative, interaction, and success, the following differences in the rules for success become apparent.[4]

Baseball Team:

- Autonomy: Very high; the individual player is the basic work unit who functions relatively independent of the other team members.
- Initiative: Team members are expected to exercise their skills only in the areas of their expertise.
- Interaction: Interactions among team members are infrequent and brief; however, each team member is aware of each other's actions.
- Success: Depends on the individual actions of each player.

Football Team:

- Autonomy: Very low; every player participates in every play.

- Initiative: Players carry out individual tasks on the basis of a coordinated, preestablished play that is carried out in a predetermined
  sequence.
- Interaction: Constant communication; team members must interact
  frequently and must communicate appropriately to fit the play at hand.
- Success: Based on an equal contribution among all team members; all
  team members must pull their own weight in the right way at the right
  time in order to produce the expected results of the play.

A self-managed rehabilitation team (SMRT) functions more like a
football team than a baseball team. The paradigm shift from a multidisciplinary
team to a SMRT is moving from being a team of stars to being a star team,
a team that manages the rehabilitation process on the following basis:

- Effective planning: The team develops a client treatment plan that is
  designed to achieve a preestablished outcome by a specified time at a
  specified cost and selects the least expensive resources to attain the
  expected outcome. The team develops a family rehabilitation plan that
  is designed to facilitate the family's ability to support the client's
  achieved outcome after discharge from rehabilitation.
- Efficient coordination: The interventions of all team members are
  carefully coordinated and sequenced across time on the basis of an
  agreed-upon individualized resource utilization plan and identified
  family needs that must be met.
- Predetermined sequence of action: The SMRT provides all services
  according to an agreed-upon individualized critical pathway, short-
  term team focus, family rehabilitation plan, and discharge plan.
- Equal contribution among all team members: All team members
  actively participate in team activities as they relate to individual
  clients or the development of the team as a whole. All team members
  proactively communicate with other team members to problem solve
  barriers to client progress and/or maintain coordination and continuity
  of services across a client's course of rehabilitation. All team members
  hold state-of-the-art knowledge and skills regarding their discipline
  and seek training from other team members in order to incorporate
  each other's goals and techniques in their discipline-specific treatment
  sessions. All disciplines document understandable and instructive
  information in timely manner.

- Constant communication: All team members continually initiate and maintain the flow of information that is required to coordinate and maintain continuity of care.

The shift from a multidisciplinary team to a self-directed interdisciplinary team requires a clear understanding on the part of both management and the team members about what a self-managed team is and how it works. Management also must be firmly committed to facilitating an environment that is conducive to the transition, as well as to providing the education and training required for the team's success.

Definition of a Self-Managed Rehabilitation Team

The concept of a SMRT is derived from the manufacturing industry's concept of self-directed work teams (SDWT). Rather than having isolated workers producing isolated parts of a product without any knowledge of or responsibility for the whole product, several manufacturers organized their workers into self-directed work teams as a means of increasing quality and reducing costs.[5] A SDWT is defined as a group of employees that is fully responsible for planning for and producing a whole product. The teams meet as frequently as necessary to coordinate work, solve problems, handle interpersonal issues, or perform administrative tasks. Any member of the team may call a team meeting. Leadership of SDWTs may vary from having no designated leader to having one elected by the team, or one assigned by management.[6]

How Does a SDWT Function?

SDWTs have the authority—delegated by management—to plan, implement, control, and improve all work processes.[7] As such, a SDWT is accountable to management for production, quality, and costs. To meet these areas of accountability, the SDWT monitors and reviews the overall process performance, scheduling, and inspecting its own work. It assigns work to group members, solves problems, and improves the work process. The SDWT, while accountable to management, is semiautonomous and is responsible for doing whatever is necessary to improve all work processes to deliver consistently a specified quantity and quality of a product within a specified time and at a defined cost as defined by management.[8] The key functions of SDWTs are directly applicable to rehabilitation teams (Exhibit 7–1).

The shift from a multidisciplinary team to a SMRT cannot be accomplished overnight or simply because management tells the team that it is now a self-managed team and leaves it up to the team to figure out what that means. To become a SMRT, the rehabilitation team must first become a high-performing interdisciplinary team. The essential components of a high-performing team are:

- Roles
  1. People clearly understand how their roles/responsibilities interrelate with those of others.

Exhibit 7–1 Key Functions of Self-Directed and Self-Managed Teams

Self-Directed Work Team	Self-Managed Rehab Team
• Consistently delivers a specified product	• Produces the expected outcome
• Delivers the product on time	• Facilitates the client's attainment of the expected outcome at or before the expected time
• Delivers the product at a cost defined by management	• Achieves the expected outcome at or below the capitated rate paid to the provider
• Monitors and controls work process performance	• Monitors client progress, ensures compliance with critical pathway, individualized resource utilization plan, and discharge plan
• Inspects its own work	• Continuously determines medical necessity and appropriate level of care
• Solves problems	• Identifies and solves barriers to client progress
• Improves the work process	• Gathers outcome data to identify areas of improvement, conducts continuous quality improvement (CQI) studies to improve process

Source: Data from M. Torres and J. Spiegel, *Self-Directed Work Teams, A Primer,* pp. 3–4, © 1990, Pfeiffer and Co.

- Activities
  1. The team produces high-quality decisions and services.
  2. The team makes decisions and produces outcomes in a timely fashion.
- Relationships
  1. The team and its individual members interact effectively with each other and with others outside the team.
  2. The team members are open in their communications with each other.
- Environment
  1. People are clear about goals for the group.
  2. Recognition and praise outweigh threats and criticism.[9]

These four essential elements (roles, activities, relationships, and environment) evolve through the process of creating a true teamwork environment. As described by Sovie:

> Teamwork requires demolishing walls between people on the team and between departments. Teamwork requires a reaching out, a bringing in and a building of bridges for easy connections. Teamwork requires a movement away from turf protection, a movement to sharing responsibilities and actions to get a quality job done.[10 (p.11)]

Team Members As Customers

The first step in demolishing walls, reaching out, and building bridges begins with an understanding that each team member is each other's customer. It begins with the acknowledgment that a team is not simply an assemblage of specialists at a team conference who report on what is occurring. The first step toward becoming a SMRT is acceptance that a true team is not a tangible entity that occurs at specified points in time but rather a continuous, interrelated, and interdependent dynamic among all members of the team—a dynamic in which each team member is committed to the provision of services that meet the expectations and needs of each other team member.

In one way or another, the ability of each team member to carry out his or her job satisfactorily depends upon how well the other team members carry out their jobs. The work activities carried out by a therapist are not solely related to the accomplishment of that therapist's job. When a product (e.g., a client outcome) is the result of the combined work activities of a number of people (e.g., rehabilitation team), the quality of the work activity of each person affects, either positively or negatively, the work activities of all others who are responsible for the production of the product. It is in this context that team members are each other's customer. That is, one team member's work is a service to another team member. If the quality of one team member's work is low, the quality of all team members who depend upon that work activity will be adversely affected. The work activity domains of communication, documentation, client care, and problem solving are critical to all team members' ability to perform their jobs in the most effective and efficient manner possible.

Communication

Clear, concise, and timely communication regarding client care concerns, education of fellow team members, and changes in the expected course of rehabilitation are of the utmost importance. All team members should be immediately informed of any concern regarding a client's physical, emotional, and/or social health, safety, and welfare. Each team member holds the responsibility to educate all other team members regarding the impact of a client's impairments, identified in their assessments, on the goals and treatment approaches of each team member. It is not unusual that the expected outcome, the client management plan, discipline short-term goals, and/or the projected discharge plan changes after the commencement of treatment. As this occurs, it is imperative that changes in a discipline's goals and treatment plan and the rationale for the change are made known to all team members in a timely manner. Similarly, recommendations regarding changes to the expected outcome or projected discharge plan should be made to the team as soon as a team member discovers clinical information indicating that such changes may be required.

Documentation

Timely dissemination of clinical information is of utmost importance. Client conferences are the typical forums for the communication of such information. It is not unusual, however, that important information arises before a scheduled conference. When this occurs, it should be entered into the client's chart rather than simply conveyed to a team member while passing each other in the hallway.

Documenting information in the chart is of vital importance to the coordination of all team members' activities. As such, it is very important that information entered into a client's chart meet the five quality criteria of being timely, legible, complete, understandable, and accurate. Documentation that meets these five criteria will be a service that enables the optimal work activities of all team members.

Client Care

Cross training is a vital service that team members can provide to each other. It will allow each discipline to reinforce the goals of all other disciplines in their treatment sessions. Adherence to the agreed-upon treatment schedule is another critical service. If one team member does not begin or end a treatment session for a given client at the agreed-upon time, the ability of all team members to provide the necessary amount of treatment to that client and, potentially, the other clients scheduled that day is decreased.

Problem Solving

Client conferences and team meetings are the primary problem-solving forums. A number of team membership responsibilities are vital to the success of such meetings. Timely attendance is critical. Identifying problems and developing solutions require that all team members hear all of the issues at the same time. Late attendance means either that the information must be repeated or that the late team member is participating in the meeting with insufficient information. Information repetition is a poor use of the time of those who were on time and insufficient information leads to inaccurate problem solutions.

Meeting Each Other's Expectations

Teamwork requires a clear understanding of what each team member expects of the other. Since expectations go beyond the surface level of what a particular team member is trained to do, it is important for the team members to discuss, explore, clarify, and agree upon the often assumed but unspoken expectations that relate to the interdependency between their functions and their ability to carry them out. Questions such as the following can help clarify the expectations team members hold of each other:

- What can you expect from me in my role? (How I see my job)
- What would I like from you to support me in my role?
- What can I expect from you?
- What would you like from me? (How you see my job)
- Which of my activities would you like more of?
- Which of my activities would you like less of?
- What additional activities do you need me to do?[11]

Meeting Team Members' Needs

The members of a team spend such a significant amount of time together, that, in a sense, they become like a second family. Thus a team, like a family, is the major source from which its members seek to meet their professional and interpersonal workplace needs. The degree to which the team as a whole meets the needs of its individual members dictates the degree to which the team is able to break down the walls between individuals and departments and build bridges to one another. Bradshaw identified the following needs that one seeks to have met by one's family:

- a sense of worth
- a sense of productivity
- a sense of relatedness
- a sense of structure
- a sense of responsibility
- a sense of affirmation
- a sense of challenge and stimulation[12]

The needs that one seeks to have met by family are strikingly similar to the following "psychological needs" of team members identified by Mallory:

- the need to contribute to the project
- the need to feel competent
- the need to achieve results
- the need to have one's efforts recognized and rewarded[13]

Bradshaw further states that: "A healthy family is one in which all members cooperate with each other to meet the collective needs of the family unit and the individual needs of each member. It strives to meet the emotional needs of each and is the growth unit, the place where the attainment of self-esteem takes place."[14]

While these concepts of family dynamics are not usually thought of in terms of teamwork, they do have applicability. The cornerstone of interdisciplinary teamwork is mutual trust, respect, and assistance. It is reasoned here that the foundation of a high-performing (healthy) team is that all members of the team cooperate to meet each other's expectations ("meet the collective needs of the family unit") and, at the same time, strive to meet the personal needs of each team member ("become the growth unit, the place where self-esteem takes place").

COMMUNICATION, CONFLICT RESOLUTION, AND PROBLEM SOLVING

To create the foundation upon which a high-performing team can evolve into a SMRT, all team members must refine their people skills: (1) communication, (2) conflict resolution, and (3) problem solving.

Communication

In everyday life, communicative interactions are usually initiated when one person wants another person to understand his or her needs, wants, feelings, concerns, opinions, or ideas. The underlying intent of communication in the workplace is no different than that of communication in daily life. Listening, not talking, is the basis of clear team communication. The ability to listen actively to one another, to truly understand each other, leads to mutual interdisciplinary trust, respect, and assistance. Active listening means that all members work to *understand* each other's needs, wants, feelings, concerns, opinions, and ideas. Active listening occurs when team members help another team member express his or her thoughts.[15] To do this, one must place one's own thoughts and beliefs on hold while listening to and exploring what another team member is trying to communicate. The greatest barrier to understanding what another team member means is to judge, evaluate, approve, or disapprove his or her statement from your own point of view. Conversely, the most powerful facilitator of understanding is to listen from the speaker's mental, emotional, professional, and/or social frame of reference. Active listening, then, is an attempt to extend and develop another team member's thinking rather than to judge or evaluate it. Active listening involves asking questions that are intended to probe and clarify. It involves paraphrasing and feeding back to the speaker what you believe he or she is trying to communicate. You seek to confirm the accuracy of your interpretation of the speaker's message and, if your interpretation is not completely accurate, you continue to probe and seek clarification until the speaker affirms that you now understand.

Just as the team members are responsible for listening actively, the speaker also has a number of responsibilities in a communicative transaction. According to Garner, the skills of sending effective messages include the following:

- *Own your message.* Collective phrases such as "some of us" or "most people on the team" communicate an element of fear and create a communication barrier. When you use phrases such as "I think . . ." or "In my opinion . . . ," you take responsibility for the ideas and feelings you are talking about.
- *Make your message complete and specific.* Messages that are nonspecific or out of context are difficult to understand and easily misinterpreted. Messages that contain more than one topic or that jump back and forth among several topics are very confusing. Messages that are specific, to the point, provide the entire context of the issue, and identify your assumptions and intentions are conducive to the active listening of the other team members.
- *Make your verbal and nonverbal messages congruent.* Your body posture, tone of voice, and facial expression should match the intent and content of your message.
- *Ask for feedback about whether you are getting your message across.* If not given the opportunity, listeners will usually hesitate to ask questions. They will think that they should understand what is being communicated and that no one else has the same problem understand-

ing you. Periodic questions such as "Am I being clear?" or "Am I giving you a good understanding of . . ." provide the listeners with the opportunity to ask questions and clarify what they are hearing.

- *Make the message appropriate to the listener's frame of reference.* Use words and expressions that are within the listener's frame of reference. Avoid the use of jargon or terminology specific to your specialty if it would interfere with an understanding of the message.
- *Describe the issue without judging or interpreting.* It is more effective to objectively describe all factors related to an issue than to cast personal judgments or make unfounded interpretations about it.[16]

Conflict Resolution

Good communication skills is one of the three "people skills" needed to become a SMRT. The ability to resolve conflicts either within the team or between it and other entities that it interacts with is another requisite skill. The first step in conflict resolution is to eliminate those that arise from either unspoken, unclear, or misunderstood team performance boundaries. Too often performance boundaries are not made known to team members until a conflict has occurred. This results in a very negative situation in which team members learn team boundaries only when they unknowingly cross one and a conflict occurs. This creates a poisoned team atmosphere in which team members feel they are walking in a field of buried land mines not knowing when they will next step on one. As discussed in the previous section of this chapter, it is the responsibility of the team leader and other levels of management to proactively define both individual and team boundaries. The most frequent sources of conflicts within a team are either unstated or unclear performance expectations, areas of responsibility and authority, and channels of communication. Consequently, at a minimum, boundaries must be established in these three areas and thoroughly understood and practiced by all team members.

Clarifying Performance Expectations

There are two types of performance expectations. The first type defines how each team member is to carry out his or her job. The second type is productivity standards. Many job performance expectations are discipline-specific and, as such, are established by the departments of the respective disciplines. However, the job performance areas of documentation, team operations, and team communication cross all disciplines. These areas of performance expectations should be established by the team leader in consultation with department managers. The following are example documentation, team operations, and team communication performance expectations (i.e., team boundaries).

Documentation

- Complete all documentation in accordance with specified time limits and content.
- Place all documentation in the appropriate sections of the medical record within the expected time frames.
- Document in a manner that clearly identifies measurable and functional changes.
- Provide a clinical rationale and your solution for slow or no progress or regression.
- Document toward all short-term goals in all progress reports.
- Provide clinical rationale as to why treatment was not provided for a particular short-term goal.
- Document progress toward family education and training goals, barriers to their attainment, and action steps taken to solve them.
- Document progress toward discharge plan goals, barriers to their attainment, and action steps taken to solve them.
- Document in a manner that is legible and easily readable by nontherapists.

Team Operations

- Independently track the number of authorized client visits, remaining visits in any given authorized period of treatment, treatment authorization expiration date, and progress report due date.
- Ensure that all visits are provided within the authorized period of treatment or inform the case manager a minimum of two weeks in advance of the need to seek an extension of the treatment authorization period.

- Ensure that progress reports are provided to the case manager one week prior to their due date when authorization for a new period of treatment will be requested.
- Actively participate in the development of the client management plan.
- Actively participate in follow-up client conferences.
- Actively participate in team development meetings.
- Arrive at client conferences/team development meetings on time and remain for the scheduled duration of the conference/meeting.
- Prepare information that will be needed to participate in client conferences/team development meetings prior to the conference/meeting.
- Prepare evaluation report and progress reports prior to the client conference and provide a copy to the case manager at the time of the conference.
- Independently pursue and complete assigned tasks at or before the established completion date.

Communication

- Immediately communicate concerns about client health, safety, and/or welfare to the case manager.
- Present recommended changes in the client management plan and/or discipline treatment plan at client conferences.
- Present discharge recommendations at client conferences.
- Immediately inform the case manager of any barriers to your ability to complete either evaluation reports, progress reports, and/or assigned tasks and identify action steps you have taken to eliminate the barriers.
- Resolve problems or conflicts directly with the individuals involved.
- Ensure that inter/intradisciplinary problems or client/family problems are resolved expeditiously.
- Present problem or conflict to the appropriate manager if it has not been resolved between the principals.
- Engage in an open and positive problem-solving style of communication with team members, client, and family.
- Communicate with each other, client, and family in a manner that is supportive of each other's efforts.

Clarifying Areas of Responsibility and Authority

To function effectively, team members must have a clear understanding of the activities each is responsible to provide as well as how and when they are to provide them. Appendix 7–A provides an example of responsibility delineation. In this example, responsibilities are established for the major activities that occur across the entire rehabilitation process. This manner of communicating by areas of responsibility is far more effective than department-specific policy and procedures. While departments must have their respective policies and procedures, they only provide discipline-specific responsibility guidelines. Team members need to know who is responsible for what throughout the entire rehabilitation process without having to read each department's policies and procedures. A document such as the one shown in Appendix 7–A is a convenient way of meeting this need. While team members hold certain responsibilities, they do not all hold the authority to make decisions in all of their areas of responsibility. A clear understanding of decision-making authority is essential to a well-organized team that is capable of providing highly coordinated services with excellent continuity of care. Exhibit 7–2 presents examples of decision-making authority. The left side lists the possible decisions involved in the day-to-day team operations and the right side of the exhibit indicates those who are authorized to make the decision. In this exhibit, MD denotes the physician, CM is the case manager, and TEAM stands for the collective decision-making by the team with the physician and the case manager included as members of the team but not the sole decision makers. DISCIPL stands for the individual therapy disciplines and REHAB TECH denotes aide or technician members of the team.

An example of a focused goal includes comparing the effectiveness and efficiency scores for a diagnostic group with national, regional, and local effectiveness and efficiency scores.

It will be noted in this example (Exhibit 7–2) that the decision-making authority for several types of decisions (items 7, 8, 9, 10, 12, 13, and 16) that are traditionally thought of as areas of discipline decision-making authority, require a team rather than a discipline decision. This approach does two things. It facilitates true interdisciplinary functioning in that it recognizes that a decision made by one team member holds the potential to

Exhibit 7–2 Examples of Decision-Making Authority

AREAS OF DECISION-MAKING AUTHORITY

DECISION	MD	CM	TEAM	DISCIPL	REHAB TECH
1. Admission to rehab. program	X				
2. Discharge from rehab. program	X				
3. Change orders	X				
4. New orders	X				
5. Approve medical consultant	X				
6. Approve nonphysician consultant (neuro psych., psych., voc., etc.)	X				
7. Identify impairments/disabilities			X		
8. Establish/modify rehabilitation outcome			X		
9. Establish/modify client treatment plan			X		
10. Establish/modify discipline goals			X		
11. Establish/modify discipline tx plan			X		
12. Establish/modify type, frequency, duration of tx		X	X		
13. Establish/modify treatment priorities			X		
14. Establish/modify treatment schedule			X		
15. Establish/modify fam. educ./trng.prog.			X		
16. Establish/modify discharge plan			X		
17. Determine when team goal has been met			X		
18. Determine when client outcome is met			X		
19. Schedule Team Conference/Team Mtg.		X		X	
20. Resolve inter/intra discipline problems		X		X	
21. Communicate with payer		X			
22. Communicate with physician		X	X	X	
23. Communicate with team members		X	X	X	X

affect the course of treatment provided by all other members. Second, because this approach vests so much decision-making authority in the team, it is a major step toward creating a self-managed team. Placing the authority to make decisions in these areas does not mean that the individual disciplines no longer make these decisions as they have in the past. What it does mean is that a discipline's decision must come to the team for discussion and possible modification prior to its implementation.

Establishing Measurable Performance Goals

Productivity standards, the second type of performance expectation, can be divided into immediate, short-term, and annual productivity goals. Immediate productivity goals are those that relate to daily or weekly productivity expectations. These are usually expressed as an expected number of units of service (UOS) or visits per day or an average number of UOS or visits per week. An example of a short-term productivity expectation would be the achievement of a preset LOS efficiency or charge efficiency score on the quarterly UDSMR report (described in Chapter 5) for a specified diagnostic group. The following are examples of annual productivity expectations:

- the percentage of clients in specified diagnostic categories that is expected to attain the predicted outcome
- the percentage of clients in specified diagnostic categories that is expected to attain the predicted outcome at or the predicted length of treatment
- the percentage of clients in specified diagnostic categories that is expected to attain the predicted outcomes at or below the expected cost
- the percentage of customers that indicates that the services received exceeded expectations

Clarifying Channels of Communication

The third source of conflicts within a team or between the team and other entities it interacts with is the lack of understanding of what information is to be communicated to whom. The locus of decision-making authority dictates to whom the communication must flow. It is incumbent upon every team member to ensure that all information required to make a decision flows to the person and/or place where the authority is vested for that decision. The identification of decision-making authority, as shown in Exhibit 7–2, simultaneously delineates the appropriate flow of communication.

Communication Breakdown

Conflict also arises when the self-interests, goals, perceptions, and values of one team member are not understood by other team members. In essence, conflict is the result of a breakdown in communication. The dynamics of shifting from a multidisciplinary team to a SMRT are such that communication breakdowns are inevitable and, therefore, conflict will occur. Further, the ability to resolve conflict in a positive manner is required for continuous high team performance. In the multidisciplinary team approach, it is the team leader's role to resolve conflicts and manage the team process. The team that learns the art of conflict resolution will be capable of evolving into a SMRT. The team that avoids or ignores conflict is the team that will become dysfunctional. Drawing an analogy once again between family systems and team systems, a dysfunctional team (family) is characterized by:

- a high level of anxiety
- rigid roles
- confused and covert rules
- reliance upon ridged and static systems
- pseudo-mutuality
- denial of problems
- shaming and blaming
- negative feedback loops (i.e., the forming of camps)[17]

Steps to Conflict Resolution

The proactive establishment of clear team boundaries eliminates many conflicts before they occur. These boundaries also provide the guidelines within which to resolve other sources of conflicts among team members.

Conflict resolution is the process of breaking down the barriers between people and departments and results in building bridges for the easy connections and overlapping of functions required in an interdisciplinary team approach to rehabilitation. To break down barriers and build the bridges, the team will need to learn and apply the following nine steps of conflict resolution.

Step 1. Take ownership of the fact that you are part of what is occurring, that conflict does not reside in the other person alone but rather between your interests, needs, wants, ideas, or opinions and those of another person.[18]

Step 2. Enter the conflict resolution process with a greater commitment to resolve the conflict than to being right.[19]

Step 3. Enter the conflict resolution process with the understanding that your perceptions and reactions to an issue do not come from what you know but from who you are. What you perceive as the reality of the situation is based on your beliefs and values. Conflict resolution begins when one is momentarily able to suspend beliefs and values and seek to understand the beliefs and values of the other party.

Step 4. Understand that perception is motivationally determined.
Typically, we believe that our evaluation of and response to an issue is based on a grasp and understanding of all that we need to know. We know what we know about the issue and we know what we don't know about it. Unfortunately, these usually represent only 25 percent (Figure 7–3) of what we will need to understand to participate successfully in the resolution of a conflict. The other 75 percent is found in learning what we don't know we don't know about the issue, a discovery that will occur only through active listening.

Step 5. Function on the basis of the "conditional truth."[20] That is, the position taken by any person on the team is accurate and valid for that person and in the best interest of the team. You may not initially agree with the position but do not judge it as invalid—momentarily suspend your beliefs and values and listen actively.

Step 6. Declare a moratorium.[21] Take time out to get the facts and problem solve. Encourage equal participation in the fact gathering and

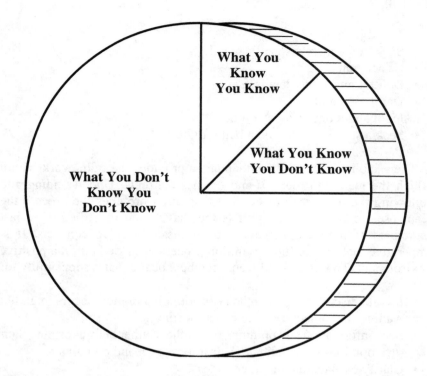

Figure 7–3 What You Don't Know Can Hurt You

problem solving. No one person owns the problem and all share the responsibility to solve it. Separate fact from opinion. Opinion usually reflects perception but not reality.

Step 7. Separate people from the problem.[22] Analyze the problem, not the people involved in it or your attitude or reaction toward the problem.

Step 8. Employ the communication skills previously described in this chapter throughout the process of conflict resolution.

Step 9. Adhere to "fair fighting rules":[23]

- Be assertive rather than aggressive.
- Stay in the now—don't drag in old issues from the past.
- Avoid lecturing.

- Avoid judgment.
- Stay with concrete specific detail.
- Be accurate.
- Don't argue about details.
- Don't assign blame.
- Fight about one thing at a time.
- Seek a solution rather than being right.[24]

The establishment of team boundaries provides the framework within which the team can identify and discuss conflicts. Understanding and following the nine steps of conflict resolution provides the process the team uses to resolve the conflicts that have been identified. One last ingredient is required, however, to successfully solve conflicts. It is imperative that the conflict resolution process is carried out in a positive environment. To this end, all team members bear equal responsibility to:

- Initiate discussions when the need for collaboration occurs (e.g., not waiting for someone else to call a meeting).
- Seek information and opinions from others either before forming their own opinions or to validate their information and opinions.
- Clarify or elaborate on others' ideas.
- Act as gatekeepers (e.g., direct conversational traffic, avoid simultaneous conversations, manage dominant talkers, and make room for reserved team members to express their views).
- Keep the discussion from digressing into nonessential minutiae.
- Seek consensus in resolving differences.
- Ease tension in the group and work through difficult matters.
- Refer to documentation and data whenever possible.
- Praise and correct others with equal fairness.
- Accept both praise and complaints.[25]

Problem Solving

A SMRT will be called upon to solve myriad problems. For example, it will be expected to participate with management in identifying appropriate measures that must be taken to reverse a decline in a program's profitability. A SMRT will also be responsible to resolve problems related to the day-to-day logistics of the rehabilitation program, quality of care issues, and customer satisfaction problems. Effective communication and conflict resolution are two of the requisite interpersonal skills that enable team members to solve problems. The following are the three problem-solving process skills that are required for effective and efficient team problem solving: (1) how to conduct a problem-solving meeting, (2) problem-solving techniques, and (3) problem-solving steps.

Problem-Solving Process Skill #1:
How To Conduct a Problem-Solving Meeting

There are five basic criteria for an effective and efficient problem-solving meeting:

1. There must be a common focus on content.
2. There must be a common group process.
3. Someone must be responsible for maintaining an open and balanced conversational flow.
4. Someone must be responsible for protecting individuals from personal attack.
5. Everyone's role and responsibility in the problem-solving process must be defined and agreed upon.[26]

The team leader is responsible for meeting the first criterion. Prior to the meeting, he or she provides all team members with an agenda and any written material that will assist in the problem-solving process. This material must be distributed in advance of the meeting to allow team members sufficient time to study it prior to the meeting. Typically, the content of problem solving focuses on potential areas of work process improvement that have been identified through the results of the team's outcome studies. Thus, the agenda identifies the specific outcome study and provides a written summary of the results and any detailed backup material, in narrative or chart form, that the group will need to identify problem(s) that, if corrected, have the greatest probability of improving the quality and efficiency of the team's services. The "interaction method" of conducting a meeting is designed to meet criteria 2 through 5.[27] In this method, there are four well-defined participant roles: (1) facilitator, (2) recorder, (3) group member, and (4) team leader.

Facilitator Role and Responsibilities

The facilitator is the neutral servant of the group and is not the team leader. He or she does not evaluate the participants' ideas nor contribute his or her own opinions or ideas regarding the problem. The group empowers the facilitator to present the problem and possible ways of attacking it and to facilitate consensus decisions regarding the nature of the problem and how it should be solved rather than decisions that require compromise. Consensus decisions are win-win decisions. They are decisions that every group member can live with. They are solutions that do not compromise any strong convictions of needs. They may not be the best solution, but team members can accept them without feeling that they are losing anything important.[28] The facilitator is also empowered to act as the groups' traffic cop. In this role, the facilitator keeps the group on track and focused on the problem to be solved, makes sure everyone has an equal opportunity to be heard, and protects each person from personal attack.

Recorder Role and Responsibilities

The recorder is also the neutral servant of the group and is the creator of the group's short-term and long-term memory. The recorder does not offer opinions or ideas related to the problem. The recorder creates the group's short-term memory by writing down on large pieces of paper in full view of the group the main points of what is said, using the words of the group members. As these key points unfold, the recorder places the sheets of paper on the walls of the room so that the group members can refer back to them as the meeting proceeds. The recorder creates the group's long-term memory by saving the sheets of paper containing the key points and either redisplaying them at subsequent meetings if the problem has not been solved or recording the group's decisions and action steps if the problem has been solved.

Group Member Role and Responsibilities

The group member is the active participant and is responsible for arriving at the meeting prepared to discuss the written material provided in advance. The group members are responsible for contributing ideas as well as for actively listening to the ideas of others. The group member is also responsible for keeping the facilitator and recorder in their neutral roles and ensuring their key points are recorded accurately.

Team Leader Role and Responsibility

The team leader sets the agenda, the purpose, and goal of the meeting and the time constraints within which the problem is to be solved. The team leader is an active participant in the same manner as any other group member but does not run the meeting. The team leader argues for his or her point of view but this does not carry any greater or lesser weight than any other member of the group. The team leader can regain control of the process and redirect it if it is not achieving its purpose and goal in a timely manner. The team leader also represents the group in meetings with other groups that are either working on the same problem or have been identified as related to the problem the group is working on.

Exhibit 7–3 presents a questionnaire that can be used to evaluate the degree to which a meeting has met the five criteria for effective problem-solving meetings from the perspective of the participants. Responses to this questionnaire can offer valuable insight for the team leader and meeting facilitator when structuring future meetings.

Problem-Solving Process Skill #2: Problem-Solving Techniques

A team may choose to use one of the following three commonly used problem-solving techniques: (1) brainstorming, (2) multivoting, and (3) nominal group technique.[29]

Brainstorming is used to ensure that all team members have an opportunity to express their point of view regarding a given problem. The brainstorming technique does not restrict ideas and, therefore, allows team members to be as creative as possible. It is also one of the easiest ways to generate a list of potential solutions to a problem.

Multivoting is a technique that is often used after brainstorming or the nominal group technique in order to reduce a long list of ideas to the few that the group believes are the most relevant to solving the problem at hand.

The nominal group technique is effective when all or some group members are new to each other, when the issue is highly controversial, or when a team is stuck in disagreement during the brainstorming or multivoting techniques.

Exhibit 7–3 Meeting Evaluation Form

Meeting: _____

Date: _____

Time _____ to _____

Circle one number for each statement. (1. Not acceptable, 2. Acceptable, 3. Good, 4. Very Good, 5. Excellent)

I understood the purpose of the meeting.	1	2	3	4	5
I had enough time to prepare for the meeting.	1	2	3	4	5
I understood what was expected of all participants.	1	2	3	4	5
Everyone expressed their ideas.	1	2	3	4	5
Everyone listened to each other's ideas.	1	2	3	4	5
Everyone understood each other's ideas.	1	2	3	4	5
All avenues of thought were clearly explored.	1	2	3	4	5
The meeting achieved its purpose and the agenda was followed.	1	2	3	4	5
My time was well spent.	1	2	3	4	5

Brainstorming Technique

General Sequence of Events: Facilitator reviews the topic, defining the subject, scope, and focus of the brainstorming session and then frames the subject in the form of a question. For example, "How can we transfer right CVA clients from inpatient acute rehabilitation to home-based rehabilitation within 10 days?" The facilitator gives everyone a minute or two of silence to think about the problem. The facilitator invites everyone to call out their ideas. The recorder records them.

Brainstorming Rules

Everyone is encouraged to put forward as many ideas as they can think of, even if they think an idea is silly. No judgment of ideas is allowed. No one is allowed to criticize another's idea, not even through nonverbal communication such as groaning or eye rolling. No discussion is allowed at this time. You can hitchhike-build upon other's ideas. All ideas are recorded on the flip chart.

Multivoting Procedure. The procedures for using a multivoting process are as follow:

1. The facilitator numbers all ideas on the sheets of paper.
2. With the author's and group's agreement, the facilitator and members of the group combine ideas that are similar.
3. Ideas are renumbered after step 2.
4. All members write down the numbers of several ideas they would like to discuss. Each member can choose a number of ideas equal to one-third of the entire list.
5. The facilitator tallies the group members' votes either by show of hands or by collecting their written votes.
6. The facilitator eliminates those items with the fewest votes.
7. The facilitator repeats steps 3 through 6 for the remaining ideas until only a few ideas remain.

Nominal Group Technique. The nominal group technique has two parts. The first part is a formalized brainstorm and the second part is selecting a solution. During a formalized brainstorm, the following steps are followed:

1. The facilitator describes the purpose of the discussion and the rules and procedures of the technique (same as brainstorming).
2. The facilitator introduces and clarifies the question and places the question in writing on the wall so all can refer back to it during the meeting. Group members are encouraged to ask questions at this time to help clarify the question. The facilitator, however, must not let this become a group discussion of the issue itself.
3. Team members generate ideas. Each team member writes down ideas in silence. No discussion, joking, or moving around is allowed. Those who finish before the others must wait quietly until everyone has finished.
4. Members next read a list of ideas. The facilitator determines how much time will be allocated to this step. Each participant reads one idea off his or her list and the recorder writes it down for all to see. The facilitator continues in a round-robin fashion until everyone's list of ideas has been recorded or until time runs out.

5. The facilitator next asks if anyone has questions or needs clarification about any of the ideas that have been recorded and displayed. At this time, the facilitator may, with the permission of the originators of the ideas, change the wording of an idea for greater clarity. When there are no more questions, the facilitator, with the permission of the ideas' originators, condenses the list as much as possible by combining ideas that are similar or redundant.

The second part of the nominal group technique involves selecting a solution. The facilitator asks team members if anyone would like to withdraw an idea they offered after they have had the opportunity for discussion and clarification. Only the author of an idea can delete an idea. The team then undertakes the multivoting technique.

Whichever technique the team chooses, the major goal and responsibility of the facilitator and each team member is to reach a consensus about what the problem is and how best to resolve it. Again, consensus is finding a proposal that all team members can support; that no member opposes. Consensus is usually not a unanimous vote; it may not represent everyone's first priorities. Consensus is definitely not arrived at through a majority vote procedure. When a majority vote is used to identify the problem and its solution, you have created a win-lose atmosphere. The majority gets something it is happy with and the minority gets something it does not want at all.[30]

Problem-Solving Process Skill #3: The Steps Required To Solve a Problem

The greatest barrier to problem solving is the tendency of group members to confuse the identification of problem solutions with identification of the problem. When this occurs, some group members are recommending solutions before there is a clear consensus as to what the problem really is. It is the responsibility of the facilitator to keep the group focused on first identifying *what* the problem is before they generate ideas about *how* to solve it. The problem is the group's perception of the content of the problem—all of the factors the group believes contribute to it. How the problem is solved is the process the group decides to arrive at a solution. There are 10 basic steps involved in solving a problem.[31] To progress through these steps effectively and efficiently, the facilitator must help the group separate problem content from problem-solving process. The problem-solving steps include:

1. stating the problem
2. perceiving the problem
3. defining the problem
4. analyzing the problem
5. generating possible solutions
6. evaluating solutions
7. deciding which solution(s) to use
8. developing a plan
9. implementing a plan
10. monitoring success of the plan

Step 1: Stating the Problem. After reviewing all pertinent background information with the team, the facilitator frames the problem in the form of a statement such as: "The average length of stay for our right hemisphere CVA clients is 25 percent longer than our average projected length of stay," or "Case management is unable to seek reauthorization for treatment that the team requests because they are not receiving progress reports within the timelines proscribed by our documentation policy and procedures."

Step 2: Perceiving the Problem. All team members may be aware of the problem but may perceive its content (e.g., all factors causal to the problem) differently. Using either the brainstorming or nominal group process techniques, the team members state their views about the problem and its causes. Within the rules of both of these techniques and in accordance with the techniques of active listening and conflict resolution, each person's perceptions are valid for that person.

Step 3: Defining the Problem. Using the multivoting process, the team reduces its list of ideas regarding the content of the problem to the fewest possible. It then reaches a consensus about the definition of the problem that the team will solve. Once consensus is achieved, the definition of the problem is stated in the form of a question. For example: "What must we do to transfer the majority of our right CVA clients from inpatient rehabilitation to home health rehabilitation within 10 days from admission?" or "What must we to do to comply with the policy and procedure guideline for entering progress reports in the chart?"

Step 4: Analyzing the Problem. Problem analysis is the first step in identifying potential solutions. Using either the brainstorming or the nominal group technique, the facilitator guides the team through the process of breaking the problem down into component parts and examining them together.

To do this, the team examines the problem in relation to the following questions:[32]

- Who is/is not involved?
- What is/is not happening?
- When is it/is it not happening?
- Where is it/is it not happening?
- Why is it/is it not happening?
- How is it/is it not happening?

Step 5: Generating Possible Solutions. Again using either the brainstorming or nominal group process, the team members offer their views as to the most effective and efficient solutions to the problem. To do this, the facilitator posses questions such as:

- What do we want the service delivery process to be when we are finished?
- What do we want it to do when we are finished?
- What should its structure be?
- What should its content be?
- Who should be involved?
- How should they be involved?
- When should they be involved?
- What should they do?

Step 6: Evaluating Solutions. Using the multivoting process, the team seeks consensus on the following questions: Are there natural categories of solutions?, Are certain categories more important than others?, Are certain solutions more important than others?, and What are the advantages and disadvantages of each?

Step 7: Deciding Which Solution(s) To Use. The team finds solutions on which it can agree, and strives for consensus—arriving at a solution that does not *compromise* any strong convictions or needs; a solution that all can accept.

Step 8: Developing a Plan. In this step, the team generates a list of all activities that will need to be performed in order to implement the solution. The list of activities is created in the form of a flowchart that indicates what the activity is, when the activity is to begin and end, where the activity is to be done, who is responsible to carry out the activity, and how the activity is to be carried out.

Step 9: Implementing the Plan.

Step 10: Monitoring Success of the Plan. The team appoints an individual or group of individuals to monitor the effectiveness of the plan. It also establishes the length of time the plan will be monitored. The results of the plan are brought back to the team at the end of that time in order to decide whether the plan should remain in effect as is or whether it needs to be modified. The Work Group Effectiveness Evaluation Form (Exhibit 7–4) can be used help the team evaluate its problem-solving process and identify areas for improvement.

THE TRANSITION FROM A HIGH-PERFORMING INTERDISCIPLINARY TEAM TO A SELF-MANAGED REHABILITATION TEAM

The MORsystem provides the framework and processes to undertake the paradigm shift from a multidisciplinary team to a high-performing interdisciplinary team to a SMRT. Using this system as the framework for clinical decision making and work process improvement, team members work to master their communication, conflict resolution, and problem-solving "people" skills. As the team members gradually master their people skills, the team leader gradually makes the transition from the traditional team leader role and responsibilities to the new roles and responsibilities of leader, coach, business analyzer, barrier buster, facilita-

Exhibit 7–4 Work Group Effectiveness Evaluation Form

1. Strongly Disagree	
2. Disagree	
3. Neither Agree nor Disagree	
4. Agree	
5. Strongly Agree	

Group: _____   Date:_____

For each statement circle a number.

I understand the purpose and goals of the group.	1	2	3	4	5
I understand the group's procedures.	1	2	3	4	5
I understand what I am expected to contribute.	1	2	3	4	5
Members of the group are comfortable with each other and understand each other.	1	2	3	4	5
Everyone speaks directly and to the point.	1	2	3	4	5
We listen carefully to each other's ideas.	1	2	3	4	5
The group's actions and activities contribute to achievement of its goals.	1	2	3	4	5
My time is well spent in this work group.	1	2	3	4	5
I am committed to the group and its success.	1	2	3	4	5

tor, customer advocate, and living example (described at the beginning of this chapter). Concurrently, as the team members refine their people skills, they leave their traditional discipline-specific roles and responsibilities and move into their new roles of customer advocate, team resource, skilled worker, team player, decision maker, problem solver, and trainer. When the team leader and team member transitions have occurred, the MORsystem provides the new paradigm (e.g., the boundaries of actions and activities and requirements to be successful within those boundaries) within which the team assumes the following self-management responsibilities of planning, implementing, controlling, monitoring, and improving its work flow.[33]

Planning

The planning functions of a SMRT include the following activities:

- Establish the client's expected outcome.
- Identify client/family goals and expectations.
- Identify risk factors.
- Identify client-specific disabilities that must be reduced.
- Establish the client's individualized resource utilization plan.
- Establish the client's individualized critical pathway.
- Establish the short-term team focus.
- Establish the family rehabilitation plan.
- Establish the preliminary discharge plan.
- Establish team members' work schedule.

Implementing

The SMRT engages in the following activities:

- Implements the client treatment plan
- Implements the family rehabilitation plan
- Implements team members' work schedule
- Interviews and selects new team members
- Implements new team member orientation and training plan

Controlling/Monitoring

The SMRT conducts the following oversight activities:

- Monitor client progress to determine medical necessity for rehabilitation.
- Monitor client progress to identify and problem solve barriers to progress.
- Monitor client progress to determine if or when the individualized resource utilization plan should be modified.
- Monitor client progress to determine when the short-term team focus should be changed.
- Monitor progress toward and update discharge plan.

- Monitor client progress to determine appropriate level of care.
- Monitor effectiveness of family rehabilitation plan.
- Monitor team member work schedule and modify as needed.
- Monitor appropriateness, effectiveness, and efficiency of team members' treatment.
- Monitor completeness and timeliness of team members' documentation.
- Monitor staffing level to ensure sufficient staff to support team responsibilities.
- Monitor team productivity to ensure it meets established standard.
- Monitor costs to ensure that they meet established standard.

Improving

The SMRT will engage in the following activities as a means to improve its work flow:

- Evaluate results of clinical, customer satisfaction, and financial studies and identify areas for improvement.
- Establish and implement a quality improvement plan related to the identified area of needed improvement.
- Monitor the effectiveness of the quality improvement plan.
- Participate in team member performance appraisals.
- Participate in team member promotion decisions.

The paradigm shift from a multidisciplinary team to a SMRT does not happen overnight. It usually occurs in the following seven phases of "shift in power" from supervisor to the team:

1. Team leader decides/announces decisions.
2. Team leader presents decision, subject to change through team feedback.
3. Team leader presents problem, asks for ideas, and then makes the decision.
4. Team selects and organizes own work; reports results to team leader.

5. Team takes responsibility for productivity and quality.
6. Team is responsible for most cost and personnel functions.
7. Team is fully autonomous.[34]

GOOD MANAGEMENT IS THE KEY TO SUCCESS

To become a self-managed rehabilitation team and maintain such a high level of function, the team must feel empowered by management. To create and maintain a sense of empowerment, management must take six steps. It must:

1. Establish clear team boundaries and the rules for success within them.
2. Establish clear and measurable performance goals and expected results.
3. Continually provide direction by identifying areas of needed change and the means to measure success in facilitating change.
4. Eliminate confusion by mutual problem solving that continually improves work process effectiveness and efficiency.
5. Continually provide knowledge, skills training, and state-of-the-art information, materials, and equipment.
6. Continually nurture interdependence through management decisions and actions that maintain team members' self-esteem, as well as by listening and responding with empathy and asking for the team's help.

Rehabilitation is a service industry. The therapists individually and the team collectively who provide the services are the key to the rehabilitation provider. The provider that does not recognize this reality will not survive. It will have high staff turnover, which will result in low quality of care. Low quality, (i.e., poor outcomes) will result in loss of contracts. Those providers who understand that their staff are the key to their success will thrive. These providers will offer their staff both the tools and a work environment that will allow them to be successful. The questionnaire, Checking Your Empowerment[35] (Exhibit 7–5) can provide a quick assessment of the degree to which a team feels empowered. The Assessing Empowerment Questionnaire (Appendix 7–B) can be used to identify specific areas that require problem solving.[36]

Exhibit 7–5 Checking Your Empowerment Level

Here are some signs of an unempowered workplace. How many do you find in your workplace? Put a check mark ✓ next to them.
- ❏ People aren't very excited about their work.
- ❏ People feel very negative.
- ❏ People only do what they are supposed to do.
- ❏ Nobody says what is on their mind.
- ❏ People are suspicious.
- ❏ People aren't willing to help out.

Unempowered employees have the following feelings. Check those that apply to your workplace.
- ❏ They don't matter.
- ❏ They should keep their ideas to themselves.
- ❏ They "rent" their job.
- ❏ Not much of their skills and energy are needed.

Empowered employees have the following feelings. Check those that apply to your workplace.
- ❏ They feel they make a difference.
- ❏ They are responsible for their results.
- ❏ They are part of the team.
- ❏ They can use their full talents and abilities.
- ❏ They have control over how they do their jobs.
- ❏ They take initiative.

Source: Reprinted with permission. *Empowerment*, Scott and Jaffee, Crisp Publications. 1200 Hamilton Court, Menlo Park, California 94025.

CONCLUSION

As rehabilitation moves into the era of managed care, the role and responsibilities of the rehabilitation team will change dramatically. As discussed in Chapter 2, provider profitability in a capitated reimbursement system will only be achieved through cost containment. Because clinical decisions drive the cost of rehabilitation, management will, of necessity, look to the team to manage its costs. In a managed care environment, the team must be able to produce an optimal client outcome while simultaneously managing its resources, service delivery format, duration of treatment, and the appropriate level of care. To be effective, quality and cost management must happen in the now (i.e., during the day-to-day provision of services). Only a self-managed rehabilitation team can meet these new responsibilities. A team cannot magically become a SMRT, however, simply by management telling it that it is one. Management must provide the team with the training, tools, and support discussed in this chapter to empower its transition from a multidisciplinary team to a high-performing interdisciplinary team and then, ultimately, to a SMRT.

REFERENCES

1. W. Belgard et al., Unpublished marketing piece (Hillsborough, OR: Belgard, Fisher, and Rayner), 1–2.
2. Belgard, 1.
3. A. Condeluci, *Interdependence: The Route to Community* (Orlando, FL: Paul M. Deutsch Press, 1991), 43–84.
4. M. Torres and J. Spiegel, *Self-Directed Work Teams: A Primer* (San Diego: Pfeiffer and Co., 1990), 3–4.
5. M. Gozzo, *Self-Directed Work Teams* (San Diego: San Diego State University and Professionals for Technology Associates, 1992), 93.
6. Gozzo, *Self-Directed Work Teams*, 21.
7. Torres and Spiegel, *Self-Directed Work Teams*, 15–26.
8. Torres and Spiegel, *Self-Directed Work Teams*, 3–4.
9. M. Sovie, Care and Service Teams: A New Imperative, *Nursing Economics 10*, no. 2 (1992) 94–125.
10. Sovie, Care and Service Teams, 11.
11. J. Neubauer, Redesign: Managing Role Changes and Building New Teams, *Seminars for Nurse Managers 1*, no. 1 (1993) 26–32.
12. J. Bradshaw, *Bradshaw On: The Family* (Deerfield Beach, FL: Health Communications, Inc., 1988), 41–43.
13. C. Mallory, *Team Building* (Shawnee Mission, KS: National Seminars Publications, 1989), 4–8.
14. Bradshaw, *Bradshaw On: The Family*, 53–54.
15. Gozzo, *Self-Directed Work Teams*, 21.
16. H. Garner, "Information Sharing and Communication," *in Guide to Interdisciplinary Practice in Rehabilitation*, ed. American Congress of Rehabilitation (Skokie, IL: American Congress of Rehabilitation Medicine, 1992), 113-130.
17. Bradshaw, *Bradshaw On: The Family*, 61–85.
18. W. Hendricks, *How To Manage Conflict* (Shawnee Mission, KS: National Seminars Publications, 1989), 18–19.
19. Hendricks, *How To Manage Conflict*, 18–19.
20. Hendricks, *How To Manage Conflict*, 18–19.

21. Hendricks, *How To Manage Conflict*, 18–19.
22. Hendricks, *How To Manage Conflict*, 18–19.
23. Bradshaw, *Bradshaw On: The Family*, 53–54.
24. Bradshaw, *Bradshaw On: The Family*, 61–85.
25. Mallory, *Team Building*, 4–8.
26. M. Doyle and D. Straus, *How To Make Meetings Work* (New York: Jove Books, 1976), 32.
27. Doyle and Straus, *How To Make Meetings Work*, 32.
28. Doyle and Straus, *How To Make Meetings Work*, 32.
29. P. Scholtes, *The Team Handbook: How To Use Teams To Improve Quality* (Madison: WI: Joiner Associates, Inc., 1993), 37–45.
30. Scholtes, *The Team Handbook*, 15.
31. Doyle and Straus, *How To Make Meetings Work*, 55–87.
32. Doyle and Straus, *How To Make Meetings Work*, 55–87.
33. Torres and Spiegel, *Self-Directed Work Teams*, 53–66.
34. Gozzo, *Self-Directed Work Teams*, 21.
35. Scott and Jaffe, *Empowerment*, 9.
36. Scott and Jaffe, *Empowerment*, 24–26.

Appendix 7–A
Delineating Areas of
Team Member Responsibility

CLIENT MANAGEMENT PROCESS

STEP 1: INTAKE

A) WHAT:
- Complete intake form
- Request original prescription and/or copy
- Forward intake form to business office/admitting

WHO: Intake coordinator

WHEN: Immediately upon completion of intake form and receipt of prescription

B) WHAT:
- Verify insurance benefits
- Complete insurance verification form
- Forward copy of insurance verification form and intake form to the outpatient case manager and outpatient scheduler

WHO: Business Office/Admitting

WHEN: Immediately upon verification of insurance benefits

C) WHAT:
- Obtain authorization numbers if they are missing
- Forward copy of intake and insurance verification with newly obtained authorization number to outpatient scheduler

WHO: Outpatient case manager

WHEN: Immediately upon receipt of authorization number

D) WHAT:
- Schedule client for initial evaluations
- Schedule client/family meeting with outpatient case manager and program coordinator
- Send copy of intake form to outpatient receptionist

- Send copy of intake form and appointment information to business office/admitting
  WHO: Outpatient Scheduler
  WHEN: By 4:00 PM each day
E) WHAT: Make patient chart
   WHO: Outpatient receptionist
   WHEN: Upon receipt of the intake form

STEP 2: INITIAL CLIENT EVALUATIONS

A) WHAT:
   - Schedule client evaluation with authorized disciplines
   - Contact referral source if client is deferred for lack of benefits and/or ability to pay
   - E-mail client evaluation schedule to therapists and outpatient receptionist
   WHO: Outpatient Scheduler
   WHEN: By 4:00 PM each day
B) WHAT: Print out client schedule at beginning of each day
   WHO: Therapists
   WHEN: The beginning of each day

STEP 3: CLIENT EVALUATION AND CLIENT/FAMILY MEETING WITH PROGRAM COORDINATOR AND OUTPATIENT CASE MANAGER

A) WHAT:
   - Identify current and expected level of function
   - Identify impairments, functional limitations, and/or disabilities in measurable terms
   - Establish functional, measurable, and time-framed short-term goals
   - Establish measurable and time-framed family education and training goals
   - Establish preliminary discharge plan
   - Complete Functional Assessment Measurement (FAM) form
   WHO: Therapists

WHEN: Within 48 hours of completing the evaluation

B) WHAT: Fill in the frequency and duration of treatment on the outpatient schedule form in the chart; and, the last therapist to see the patient either: (1) takes the patient and the outpatient schedule form to the outpatient scheduler, or (2) calls the outpatient scheduler to come and get the patient and the schedule

WHO: Therapists

WHEN: On the day the last therapist's evaluation is completed

C) WHAT: Dictate/write evaluation report that includes the following content:
- Client impairments and/or functional limitations stated in measurable terms
- Client disabilities stated in measurable terms
- Client goals
- Family goals
- Residential issues that may have impact on the rehabilitation program:
    1. safety
    2. physical barriers
    3. level of environmental stimulation
    4. family understanding of client's impairments, disabilities, and needs
    5. degree of family support
- Client and family education and training needs
- Projected functional outcome
- Projected frequency and duration of treatment
- Preliminary discharge plan

WHO: Therapists

WHEN: Within 72 hours of completing the evaluation

D) WHAT: Meet with client and family to:
- Describe program coordinator's role
- Describe the rehabilitation program and process
- Identify client and family goals and the barriers they believe must be reduced to reach those goals
- Discuss medical necessity criteria for continued treatment
- Discuss purpose and importance of home programs
- Discuss importance of client attending all treatment sessions

- Discuss importance of family members attending treatment sessions as much as possible

WHO: Program coordinator

WHEN: During same time period as the client evaluation

E) WHAT: Meet with client and family to:
- Describe role of outpatient case manager
- Conduct an initial case management evaluation
- Orient client and family to the logistics and physical layout of the program
- Discuss funding issues and process

WHO: Outpatient case manager

WHEN: During the same time period as the evaluation

STEP 4:   INITIAL CLIENT CONFERENCE

WHAT:	WHO:
Funding and length of stay identified	Case manager
Medical history/medications/ precautions	Program coordinator
Family status	Program Coordinator/team
Psychosocial history	Social worker/psychologist
Client/family goals identified	Program coordinator/team
Risk factors identified	Team
Identify previous level of function	Team
Identify current level of function	Team
Establish projected outcome level of function	Team
Establish projected frequency and duration of treatment	Disciplines
Establish short-term team focus	Team
Establish individualized resource utilization plan	Team
Identify cross-discipline impairment/ functional limitation/disability	Team
Establish family education/training goals	Team
Establish preliminary discharge plan that includes:	Team
• Safety issues	

- Physical barriers that must be modified
- Equipment needs
- Client/family supports that will be needed
- Additional community resources that will be needed
  WHEN: Within 72 hours of completion of client evaluation
  by all disciplines

**STEP 5: COMMUNICATION OF CLIENT TREATMENT PLAN
TO CLIENT AND FAMILY**

WHAT: Discuss client treatment plan with client and family
along with each discipline's short-term client goals, family
education and training goals, and preliminary discharge plan
WHO: All therapists and program coordinator
WHEN: Within 72 hours of the initial client conference

**STEP 6: IMPLEMENTATION OF CLIENT TREATMENT
PLAN, FAMILY EDUCATION AND TRAINING PLAN,
AND DISCHARGE PLANNING**

WHAT:
- Provide rehabilitation services that are:
  1. Specific and effective approaches to the attainment of the
     client's expected outcome level of function
  2. Specific and effective approaches to interdisciplinary team
     goals
  3. Based on a minimum of biweekly objective and subjective
     measurement of progress toward goals
- Identify causal factors for regression, slow, or no progress
  and determine whether:
  1. Treatment should continue as planned
  2. the treatment plan should be altered
  3. the goals should be modified
  4. the frequency and amount of treatment should be in-
     creased or decreased

5. the individualized service delivery plan should be altered (individual, group, dual, cotreat, aides, etc.)
6. the prognosis should be revised
7. the estimated length of treatment should be revised, and/ or
8. treatment should be discontinued

WHO: All therapists
WHEN: Beginning with the first scheduled treatment session and ongoing thereafter

STEP 7:   ONGOING THERAPY SCHEDULING

WHAT: Provide ongoing schedule changes in writing on the outpatient schedule form to outpatient scheduler
WHO: All therapists
WHEN: One (1) week prior to the end of the currently scheduled block of visits. Note: Client schedules will not be changed due to therapist schedule conflicts. If a conflict occurs (e.g., meeting called at the same time as a scheduled treatment), it is the therapist's responsibility to find another therapist to treat the client.

STEP 8:   ONGOING CLIENT AND FAMILY COMMUNICATION

WHAT:
• Identify and respond to client/family questions, concerns, or problems
• Continually inform client and family of purpose of various treatment approaches, progress toward short-term goals, and barriers to progress
• Inform program coordinator of the need for a family conference on an as-needed basis

WHO: All team members
WHEN: Ongoing from date of initial evaluation

STEP 9: FOLLOW-UP CLIENT CONFERENCE

WHAT:	WHO:
Update on funding and length of stay	Outpatient case manager
Update number of visits remaining	Team
Discuss family questions and concerns	Team
Review progress toward short-term/client/ family goals and expected outcome	Team
Problem solve and establish action plan for areas of lack of progress or regression	Team
Review progress toward short-term team focus and establish new short-term team focus	Team
Review progress toward discharge plan goals and update plan	Team
Provide outpatient case manager and program coordinator with copy of progress report	Team

WHEN: For inpatient, at least every other week. For outpatient, at least every four weeks.

STEP 10: CLIENT, FAMILY, PAYER FOLLOW-UP CONFERENCE COMMUNICATION

A) WHAT:
  • Program coordinator presents and discusses the results of the follow-up client conference with client and family
  • Each therapist reviews and discusses his or progress report information and any problem-solving information with the client and family during a regularly scheduled treatment session

  WHO: Program coordinator and therapists
  WHEN: Within 72 hours of the follow-up client conference

B) WHAT:
  • Write/dictate client progress report
  • As required, send progress report to payer
  • Verbally communicate results of follow-up client conference to payer

  WHO: Outpatient case manager
  WHEN: Within 48 hours of the follow-up client conference

STEP 11: CLIENT DISCHARGE

> WHAT: Program coordinator of therapists requests outpatient case manager to place client on conference schedule prior to discharge
> WHO: Program coordinator/therapists
> WHEN: A minimum of three weeks prior to the recommended discharge date

STEP 12: TEAM/CLIENT/FAMILY DISCHARGE CONFERENCE

> A) WHAT: Schedule discharge conference
>   WHO: Outpatient case manager
>   WHEN: Two weeks prior to the discharge date
> B) WHAT: Review progress toward all discharge goals and establish action plan for unresolved goals
>   WHO: Client, family, and all team members
>   WHEN: Two weeks prior to discharge

Appendix 7–B
Assessing Empowerment Questionnaire

Instructions

If you feel that a statement is *very true*, circle the number 1.
If you feel that a statement is *somewhat true*, circle the number 2.
If you feel that a statement is *somewhat untrue*, circle the number 3.
If you feel a statement is *very untrue*, circle the number 4.

EMPOWERMENT ASSESSMENT

1. Clarity of Purpose

People know where they stand.	1	2	3	4
I know what is expected of me.	1	2	3	4
Tasks and responsibilities are clearly organized.	1	2	3	4
Systems and procedures are adequate.	1	2	3	4
I know what the company (team) stands for.	1	2	3	4

2. Morale

People are trusted.	1	2	3	4
Policies are flexible enough to consider personal needs.	1	2	3	4
I feel respected as a person.	1	2	3	4
Individual differences in lifestyle and values are respected.	1	2	3	4
I like working here.	1	2	3	4
There is a positive spirit.	1	2	3	4
If I had a personal problem, the company (team) would stand by me while I worked it out.	1	2	3	4

3. Fairness

I approve of the things that go on here.	1	2	3	4
People are treated fairly.	1	2	3	4
I trust what the company (team) says.	1	2	3	4

Source: Reprinted with permission. *Empowerment*, Scott and Jaffe, Crisp Publications. 1200 Hamilton Court, Menlo Park, California 94025.

4. Recognition

Individual effort is rewarded appropriately.	1	2	3	4
If people do something well, it is noticed.	1	2	3	4
The company (team) looks at what you can do, not who you know.	1	2	3	4
The company (team) expects the best from people.	1	2	3	4

5. Teamwork

People help each other out.	1	2	3	4
People work together to solve difficult problems.	1	2	3	4
People care for each other.	1	2	3	4
People here are out for the company (group), not themselves.	1	2	3	4

6. Participation

People have a voice in decisions.	1	2	3	4
Problems are shared.	1	2	3	4
People get the resources they need to do their jobs.	1	2	3	4

7. Communication

I am kept informed of what's going on in the company.	1	2	3	4
Communication is clear and timely between groups.	1	2	3	4
I understand why things are asked of me.	1	2	3	4

8. Healthy Environment

People are able to manage the pressure of their work.	1	2	3	4
I am not expected to do too many things.	1	2	3	4
Change is managed well.	1	2	3	4
Red tape and procedures don't interfere with getting things done.	1	2	3	4
I am able to grow and learn.	1	2	3	4
There are opportunities for career development.	1	2	3	4

UNDERSTANDING YOUR SCORES

For each of the eight areas, average the scores by dividing your total of all the numbers you circled by the number of questions in that section. If several people in a work team take this assessment, you can also average all their responses together for a group score.

Write your average scores here for each section:
1. _____
2. _____
3. _____
4. _____
5. _____
6. _____
7. _____
8. _____

Mark your two highest scores with an asterisk (*). Circle your two lowest scores.

Generally, the sections in which the average is above 2.0 raise issues you should talk about in your team.

Which areas show a lot of difference in scores between team members? Talk about it in a group.

What can you do to make changes that will lead to a more empowered workplace?

_____
_____
_____
_____
_____

CHAPTER 8

Successful Documentation

KEY POINTS:

- Documentation must be usable, feasible, auditable, and legally defensible.

- Documentation must establish the medical necessity of treatment.

- Documentation must provide information for outcome studies.

- Documentation must provide information required for licensure and accreditation.

Successful documentation is the recording of clinical information that is usable, auditable, and legally defensible. An appropriate mindset and perception of the purpose of documentation is required to create successful documentation. Documentation is often viewed by the therapist as a necessary evil, a time-consuming task in the hectic world of service delivery.

Documentation of clinical interventions, however, is far more than a peripheral task to hands-on treatment. It is far more than a reimbursement requirement. Documenting clinical findings, goals, treatment approaches, client progress, barriers to progress, solutions to those barriers, client and family training and education, discharge plans, and the implementation of those discharge plans is a significant clinical responsibility, a client care responsibility that is equal in importance to accurate assessment and appropriate treatment. It is a critical quality and cost management tool. With respect to quality, the clinical record is the primary tool for both concurrent clinical case management and retrospective program evaluation. With respect to cost control, documentation determines prior authorization of services and payment for services after they have been rendered. Finally, therapists hold a significant professional obligation to their clients to document accurately, appropriately, completely, understandably, and in a timely manner. The absence of such can mean the decision by payers not to authorize the treatment that clients need or to authorize an inadequate frequency and duration of services. The absence of good professional documentation can also result in a payer's decision not to authorize continued treatment when it is needed to reach the client's maximum potential.

PURPOSE OF DOCUMENTATION

Clinical documentation is the process of creating a serial medical record that describes the client's condition, the course of therapeutic intervention employed to improve that condition, and the client's response to those interventions, from admission to discharge. This record serves seven purposes: (1) the therapist's "memory," (2) communication, (3) clinical case management, (4) certification, treatment authorization, and/or reimbursement, (5) a legal record, (6) licensure and accreditation, and (7) continuous quality improvement.

Therapist's "Memory"

One of the original and most fundamental reasons that health care professionals document their clinical findings, therapeutic interventions, the expected results of those interventions, and the actual results is that they cannot carry all of this information for all of their clients in their head. Because of this they "store" the information on paper or in a computer so that they can "retrieve" it whenever it is needed.

Communication

The medical record is a vital communication link between the therapist and other health care professionals who are also involved in making decisions about a client's care yet who cannot always communicate directly with each other. Documentation is also vital to continuity of care. When a primary therapist is sick or on vacation, it is the major source of information that tells the temporary therapist what the primary therapist's goals are, what specific therapy interventions are to be used in relation to each goal, and what the client's usual response is to those interventions. Documentation also sustains continuity of care when a client is transferred from one level of care to another.

Clinical Case Management

Documentation is a picture of the rehabilitation process. It describes the client's impairments and disabilities upon admission to rehabilitation, the expected outcome of rehabilitation, the short-term goals that must be met to attain that outcome, the therapeutic interventions that will be employed to achieve each of the short-term goals, and the client's response to those interventions across time. This picture provides the therapist, the team, and the internal case manager with an objective basis upon which to determine the appropriateness, effectiveness, and necessity of therapeutic intervention.

Certification/Recertification, Treatment Authorization/ Reauthorization, and Reimbursement

The therapist's documentation is the primary basis upon which an outpatient Medicare client's physician decides whether to certify the medical necessity for an initial 30-day period of therapy and then to recertify the medical necessity of continued treatment past that initial 30-day period. Medicare also retrospectively reviews the therapist's documentation to determine whether a bill for therapy services should be paid. Private health insurance payers and Medicaid also use the therapist's documentation as a basis for their decisions as to whether they will authorize the initiation of therapy and reauthorize its continuation after the initial number of visits have been used. They also use the therapist's documentation to decide how many additional visits will be authorized. Medicare does not assure reimbursement by preauthorizing therapy services. It does, however, review therapists' documentation after the services have been provided and render a decision about whether the services were medically necessary. If they are not deemed medically necessary, the Medicare claim (i.e., the bill from the provider) is "denied" and the provider is not paid.

Legal Record

The therapist's documentation, and the medical record as a whole, is a legal document. It is a legal record of a therapist's professional knowledge, judgment, skills, and actions. As such, its content can be used as evidence in legal proceedings. It can be admitted into evidence in a malpractice suit either for or against the therapist and/or the therapist's employer. The extreme importance of clear, accurate, objective, and measurable documentation can be seen in the manner in which malpractice is determined. Malpractice is typically defined as negligence or legally actionable careless treatment resulting in injury to a patient.[1] From a legal perspective, a determination of malpractice or negligence is based on four questions: (1) Did the therapist owe the client the "duty of care" (i.e., was the therapist obligated to provide the care by terms of employment, written or oral contract, licensure and/or certification)?, (2) Did the therapist "breach" that duty of care (i.e., did the therapist evaluate and treat the client in accordance with acceptable professional standards)?, (3) Was the client injured?, and (4) Was the injury the result of the therapist's "breach" of duty of care? The therapist's documentation can also be subpoenaed by a client's attorney who has filed suit against another entity. Take, for example, a personal injury case in which a client sustains a traumatic brain injury as the result of a fall in an unmarked area of wet floor in a grocery store. As a result of the brain injury, the client experiences impaired attention and concentration, short-term memory loss, and difficulty with word retrieval and balance during ambulation. In personal injury litigation, the client's attorney will use the therapist's documentation to prove that the client suffered compensable brain injury as a result of negligence on the part of the grocery store's management. On the other hand, the defendant's attorney will try to use the very same documentation to prove that the therapist's findings were inaccurate, inconclusive, or deviated from standards of professional practice. The defense attorney will contend to the jury that the therapist's findings do not substantiate the presence of brain injury.

In cases of this nature, it also is not uncommon for the therapist to be called to testify. The defense attorney will attempt to nullify the therapist's testimony by finding inconsistencies both within the documentation and between the therapist's oral testimony and his or her documentation.[2] As can be readily seen, good documentation is the cornerstone of defense against litigation involving clinical practice. In legal proceedings, the documentation must clearly and absolutely establish that the treating therapist did not deviate from the standard of care ordinarily adhered to by the therapist's profession.[3]

Licensure and Accreditation

All providers of rehabilitation services must be licensed by the state within which they provide services. The majority of providers also voluntarily seek to become accredited by the Joint Commission on Accreditation of Healthcare Organizations (Joint Commission) and/or the Commission on Accreditation of Rehabilitation Facilities (CARF). Licensure and accreditation are critical to the financial viability of providers of rehabilitation services. They cannot provide any services without a license. Accreditation is viewed by referral sources and payers as an indicator that the provider's services will be competent and of high quality. To become either licensed or accredited, a provider must meet certain practice standards. A provider's compliance with these standards is determined by an on-site review of client care practices by representatives of the licensure and accrediting bodies. These reviewers use the medical record as the primary source of information upon which to base their recommendation whether or not the provider should be licensed or accredited.

Continuous Quality Improvement

Clinical documentation provides the database required to conduct clinical effectiveness and efficiency outcome studies. The results of the outcome studies provide the rehabilitation team with the information it needs to pinpoint service delivery problem areas and conduct continuous quality improvement (CQI) studies to rectify them. The medical record, in turn, is used to abstract the data that are necessary to monitor the effectiveness of the CQI action plan. The accuracy, consistency, timeliness, and completeness of the therapist's documentation is absolutely vital to conducting valid and useful outcome studies and CQI activities. The saying used in computer data analysis, "garbage in—garbage out," is very apropos to outcome studies and CQI.

DOCUMENTATION MUST BE "USER-FRIENDLY"

Since the content of clinical documentation is used by a wide audience for a variety of reasons, it must be "user-friendly" for both the therapist who generates the client's clinical record and the potential audiences that will also use and rely upon it to carry out their jobs. To be "user-friendly," a documentation system and the content it produces should meet four criteria. It must be: (1) usable, (2) feasible, (3) auditable, and (4) legally defensible.

Usable Documentation

Usable documentation is that which is readable and understandable and supports clinical case management.

Readable Documentation

Readable documentation is that which is legible; provides only information that is pertinent to understanding the client's medical condition, problems resulting from it, and potential to benefit from therapy; and is presented in a logical sequential reporting format that does not require readers to "hunt" for needed information. For example, the format of an initial evaluation report would include pertinent history, a statement of the problem, clinical findings, projected outcome of treatment, short-term goals required to achieve that outcome, and treatment interventions that will be used to achieve those goals. The progress report format would be one that restates the expected outcome, compares the client's current status with his or her status at the beginning of the time period covered by the progress report for all short-term goals, and describes any problems that have interfered with progress toward short-term goals, actions that have been taken to alleviate the problems, and any new short-term goals.

Understandable Documentation

Understandable documentation is that which presents clinical information in language that can be understood by all who use it. It is documentation that is as free of professional jargon as possible and defines it when it must be used. It is also documentation that does not use abbreviations that are known only to the therapist or within the facility where the therapist practices. Understandable documentation is that which meets the unique interests and needs of all who may use it.

Supports Clinical Case Management

Documentation that supports clinical case management is that which allows the primary therapist, a temporary therapist, or the therapist at a client's next level of care to immediately understand the client's projected outcome, short-term goals, and specific effective treatment interventions. It is also documentation that tracks progress toward goals in a measurable and time-framed manner. Such progress reporting provides the basis upon which the current or future therapist can decide whether treatment approaches are effective, whether they should be modified, or whether continued treatment is medically necessary.

Feasible Documentation

Feasible documentation refers both to the documentation system and content. The criterion of feasible documentation is that it is not time-consuming. Feasible documentation, then, is a system and the content required by that system that minimizes staff time in producing and reviewing it without sacrificing completeness and quality. Feasible documentation also minimizes the time it takes other users to review, analyze, and understand it.

Management is responsible for creating a feasible documentation system. Today's therapists must recognize, process, and act upon large amounts of clinical, payer, and regulatory information. Clearly, the paper-based patient chart is no longer an efficient and effective means of organizing and managing patient care. The medical record, as historically structured, accessed, and used, does not meet today's need to have information available when and wherever the therapist or other documentation users are at any given moment. Feasible documentation requires an electronic information management system—a computer-based system that can be immediately accessed by the therapist at the time of the client-therapist interaction. Such a system should be driven by a single database that allows the therapist to record assessment information, select diagnoses, develop a treatment plan, write reports, and fill out charge slips and insurance forms during client-therapist interaction. In essence, to create feasible documentation, therapists will need an information management system that is capable of capturing every client-therapist interaction as it occurs and wherever it occurs, with the least expenditure of time and effort by the therapist. Such a system must also be designed in a manner that allows all other parties involved with the client to access the client's clinical documentation whenever and wherever needed.

Auditable Documentation

An audit, or review, of the medical chart may be conducted for a number of reasons and may be carried out before, during, and/or after the termination of therapy. It is the therapist's responsibility to review the medical record before initiating treatment as part of the clinical evaluation that determines the medical necessity of treatment. The therapist also reviews the medical record during the course of treatment to determine the medical necessity of continued treatment. The team or its designee performs audits of the medical record to collect data for outcome and CQI studies. Payers audit the medical record for the purpose of authorization/reauthorization of treatment or payment determinations. The medical record is used by state licensure and national accreditation bodies to determine a provider's level of compliance with its standards. The medical record may also be audited for purposes of litigation. Auditable documentation is that which allows for objective concurrent and retrospective review of a client's rehabilitation program and response to it. Auditable documentation must include objective and measurable descriptions of the client's impairments and disabilities; the expected outcome of therapy; functional, measurable, and time-framed short-term goals; a statement of treatment approaches; and objective measurement of progress across time. The documentation must also describe any unforeseen problems that arose during the course of treatment and the manner in which the problems were resolved.

Legally Defensible

Legally defensible documentation is that which meets the above criteria for readable, usable, and auditable documentation. In addition, it is documentation that is presented in a nonjudgmental and nonbiased manner.

Additionally, the documentation should not include personal conjecture, third-party information, or any negative comments about other practitioners personally or about their treatment procedures and results, or any concerns regarding the manner in which the facility is being managed. Concerns about other practitioners or management should be expressed in the proper documents and forums.

SUCCESSFUL DOCUMENTATION CONTENT

As described earlier in this chapter, successful documentation is that which is usable, auditable, and legally defensible. Different providers and different payers use a variety of documentation forms. Regardless of the type of form used, however, it is the content of the documentation that is critical. It is the content of the form that establishes the medical necessity of treatment, forms the basis of day-to-day clinical case management, provides an objective record of assessment findings and a client's response to treatment, and captures the data needed to perform outcome studies. The remainder of this chapter will present guidelines for and examples of documentation content that meet all of the criteria for successful documentation. The content of an initial evaluation and treatment plan, including effective short-term goals, will be addressed, as well as appropriate progress report information. The chapter will conclude with detailed information regarding the completion of the Medicare 700 and 701 forms.

Establishing the Medical Necessity of Treatment

The medical necessity of initiating treatment is based on seven clinical questions:

1. Does the client have a medical condition?
2. Has the medical condition resulted in a decrease in the client's ability to meet his or her usual and customary daily living needs?
3. Has the medical condition resulted in specific impairments that are causing the client's disabilities?
4. Given the type and severity of the client's impairments and disabilities, does the client hold a prognosis for making significant practical improvement?

5. If the client holds a prognosis of making significant practical improvement, are the skilled services of a therapist required to achieve it?
6. Is the treatment specific and effective to the client's condition?
7. What frequency and duration of treatment will be required?

The purpose of a therapist's initial evaluation is to answer these seven questions and the purpose of the therapist's initial evaluation report is to document those answers. If the answer to all of these questions is "yes," the therapist has established the medical necessity for skilled therapy. The results of the evaluation have established: (a) that the client has a medical condition, (b) that the medical condition has resulted in a decrease in functional daily living abilities, (c) that specific impairments related to the therapist's field of expertise exist that are causing the client's disabilities, (d) that the client has the potential to make significant practical improvement, and (e) that skilled therapy is required to facilitate that improvement. Having conducted an evaluation that produced clinical findings that support a "yes" response to the first five questions, the therapist must next document the results of the evaluation in the medical record that substantiate his or her conclusion that therapy is medically necessary. The therapist's initial evaluation report is used for this purpose.

Initial Evaluation Report

The *initial evaluation report* responds to these questions by providing information regarding the client's history, a description of his or her functional abilities before and after the medical episode, assessment results, a treatment plan, and the recommended frequency and duration of treatment that will be required to increase the client's functional abilities. Following are examples of initial evaluation report content that respond to each of the seven questions used to establish the medical necessity of treatment.

Does the Client Have a Medical Condition?

The client's medical history substantiates a "yes" response to this question. The history identifies the reason for referral to the therapist. This section of the initial evaluation report should only contain information that has a direct relationship to and bearing on the diagnosis, prognosis, goals, treatment plan, and/or the client's potential for progress. It should contain the primary medical diagnosis (e.g., stroke [CVA], traumatic brain injury [TBI], spinal cord injury [SCI], etc.) and the date of its occurrence. It should also contain any other medical diagnoses or risk factors that will help others understand the therapist's decisions regarding the expected outcome of treatment, the treatment plan, and the recommended frequency and duration of treatment.

An example of a medical diagnosis is a patient who incurred right CVA on 1/28/98. CT 1/29/98 showed right temporo-occipital infarction. Patient has a reactive depression and a premorbid history of hypertension and dizziness.

Has the Client's Medical Condition Resulted in a Decrease in the Client's Ability To Meet His or Her Usual and Customary Daily Living Needs?

A "yes" response to this question is substantiated in the initial evaluation report by a description of the client's level of function prior to the medical episode and a description of his or her current (i.e., at the time of the evaluation) level of function.

Prior Level of Function. This is a description, stated in measurable terms, of the degree of independence with which the client carried out his or her personal, household, community, work/avocational/educational, and leisure daily living activities before the onset of the medical episode.

Current Level of Function. The current level of function is a statement that describes, in measurable terms, the client's degree of independence in carrying out his or her personal, household, community, work/avocational/ educational, and leisure daily living activities after the onset of the medical episode.

This statement is one of the most critical elements in the initial evaluation report. The client's level of function, not the type and severity of his or her impairments, per se, is the therapist's and payer's sole determinant of the medical necessity of treatment. The purpose of treatment is not simply to reduce the client's level of impairment, but to reduce his or her level of disability. Consequently, the medical necessity of initiating treatment is not based on the severity of a client's impairments but rather on the extent of his or her disability. The extent of disability is determined by the degree of gap between the client's previous and current level of functioning. The client's current level of functioning also establishes the baseline from which functional progress will be measured once treatment begins. Thus, the measurement and description of the client's prior and current level of function is also critical to determining the medical necessity of continued treatment. For this reason, this section of the evaluation report must identify, in measurable terms, specific areas of personal, household, community, work/avocational/educational, and leisure disability. Typically, degree of disability is measured and stated in one of two ways: (1) in terms of the degree of assistance required from another, or (2) in terms of the degree to which the client can perform a daily living activity. Level of assistance is usually measured by terms such as totally dependent, maximum assistance, moderate assistance, minimal assistance, standby assistance, modified independent, and independent or the degree to which the client can perform a particular daily living skill. Degree of client performance is usually expressed in the form of a percentage (e.g., the client can perform 50 percent of upper body dressing, the client can accurately communicate 60 percent of his personal care needs). An example of prior level of function would be a client, who prior to CVA, was independent in all personal, household, community access, and leisure activities of daily living (ADLs). The current level of functioning for the same client would be such that he requires moderate assistance for his personal and household ADLs and maximum assistance for his community access and leisure ADLs.

Has the Medical Condition Resulted in Specific Impairments That Are Causing the Client's Disability?

A "yes" answer to this question is supported by the results of the therapist's assessment. The assessment results section of the initial evaluation report identifies the type and severity of impairments that are contributing to the disabilities described in the Current Level of Function section. This section describes the tests and/or evaluation procedures that were used and the results of these assessments stated in measurable terms. The following are examples of assessment results for physical therapy, speech-language pathology, and occupational therapy.

Physical Therapy Assessment Results. Client presents with mild decrease in left upper and lower extremity strength, poor dynamic standing balance, and a moderate decrease in upper and lower extremity control secondary to moderate proprioceptive impairment.

Speech-Language Pathology Assessment Results. Client presents with mild dyspraxia; mild written language impairment; and moderate attention, short-term memory, and problem-solving impairments.

Occupational Therapy Assessment Results. Client presents with moderate decrease in dynamic sitting balance, absent right upper extremity coordination and strength, moderate right-hand edema, and moderate to severe decrease in right upper extremity proprioception.

Given the Type and Severity of the Client's Impairments and Disabilities, Does the Client Hold a Prognosis of Making Significant Practical Improvement?

A "yes" answer to this question is substantiated in the therapist's statement of the expected outcome of treatment. The expected outcome describes *what* the therapist believes the client will be able to do as a result of his or her treatment that the client was unable to do prior to treatment. The following are examples of expected outcomes for physical therapy, occupational therapy, and speech-language pathology.

Physical Therapy. Within 18 visits, the client will be able to ambulate safely with a single-point cane on all surfaces in order to be modified independent in all personal ADLs, and a decreased type and amount of his usual and customary household, community access, and leisure ADLs.

Occupational Therapy. Within 18 visits, the client will be modified independent in all self-care, meal preparation, and light housework.

Speech-Language Pathology. Within 24 visits, the client will be independent in communicating all personal ADL needs, will need standby assistance in communicating household ADL needs, and minimal assist to communicate community ADL needs.

What Are the Special Circumstances Regarding Prognosis?

Certain clients require additional documentation to that described above to substantiate the medical necessity of treatment. Typical special circumstances that require such additional documentation include:

- cases in which a long period of time has passed between the onset of the medical condition and the current intent to initiate treatment and

the client has received no previous treatment
- cases similar to the one above, except that the client has previously received treatment
- progressive neurologic diseases and metastatic carcinoma

In the case of the client who is seeking to begin treatment after a longer than usual period of time since onset, the therapist must document why treatment was not initiated earlier and why it is reasonable to expect its institution at this time is reasonable and necessary to the client's condition. For example, there may have been recent positive changes in the client's medical, emotional, cognitive, and/or family status that precluded treatment in the past. These may also be reasons why therapy was previously discontinued. Their alleviation now indicates that the resumption of treatment is reasonable and necessary. Finally, newly developed treatment techniques, treatment equipment, and/or assistive technology that was not available in the past may support the medical necessity of treatment both for the client who previously received no therapy and for the one who did.

Clients with progressive neurologic diseases or incurable metastatic carcinoma require a different type of documentation to support the medical necessity of treatment. Unfortunately, clients in these two categories are not on a rehabilitation track in which treatment is expected to increase and stabilize a higher level of functional abilities. The expectation in these cases is that treatment will assist the client to compensate for his or her level of impairment and, therefore, be able to better utilize his or her existing abilities. Consequently, to support the medical necessity of treatment of these clients, the documentation must reflect that the client has the perceptual and cognitive abilities to participate in treatment and it must reflect goals and a treatment plan that are oriented toward facilitating better use of existing abilities and establishing a maintenance plan of care. The frequency and duration of treatment would typically be one to two weeks, two to three times a week. Finally, since clients in these diagnostic categories typically experience a decrease in functional abilities across time, some quite rapidly and some over a period of many years, the documentation should also include the signs and symptoms that would necessitate reevaluating the client so that the previous compensatory techniques and maintenance plan of care can be modified to match the client's new level of impairment.

Is the Treatment Specific and Effective to the Client's Condition?

The content of the treatment plan establishes that treatment is specific and effective to the client's condition. To do so, the treatment plan must include the expected outcome (long-term goal) of treatment, the short-term goals that must be achieved across time to attain the expected outcome, the type of treatment procedures that will be employed to achieve the short-term goals, the family training goals, the frequency and duration of treatment, and the discharge plan.

Expected Outcome (Long-Term Goal). The stated expected outcome must relate to the disabilities identified in the "current level of function" section of the initial evaluation report.

Short-Term Goals. The statement of the client's current level of function is the critical data element used to determine the medical necessity for initiating treatment. Short-term goals are the critical data elements used to determine the medical necessity of continued treatment. The client's rate and degree of progress toward the achievement of short-term goals is used to measure whether or not the client is making significant practical improvement. Short-term goals are directly related to the expected outcome and delineate the sequence of activities or events that must occur in specific impairments, functional limitations, and/or disabilities in order to attain the expected outcome. To objectively determine whether a client is making significant practical improvement, a short-term goal must be measurable and time-framed (instructions for writing short-term goals is discussed in detail later on in this chapter). Exhibit 8–1 presents an example of short-term goals for occupational therapy, physical therapy, and speech-language pathology. Consider which of these could be used to objectively determine whether a client has made significant practical improvement.

Treatment Procedures. Treatment procedures describe the activities, procedures, and/or modalities that will be used. They should identify assistive and adaptive equipment as well as any orthotics and/or prosthetics that will be used in the course of treatment. In the case of an inpatient, the treatment procedures should also include any procedures that will be taught to the family. In the case of an outpatient, they should include the client's home exercise program. The home program should describe the

Exhibit 8–1 Example of Short-Term Goals

Speech-Language Pathology
1. Increase word retrieval in all communication environments
2. Decrease auditory comprehension impairments so client can answer yes/no questions with 90% accuracy
3. Increase problem-solving skills to 90% accuracy in 4 weeks to enable client to respond accurately to emergency situations with standby assist 100% of the time

Occupational Therapy
1. Client to doff/don clothes
2. Improve passive range of motion (PROM) of right upper extremity (RUE) 10° and active range of motion (AROM) 50°
3. Increase right shoulder AROM to within functional limits in 3 weeks to enable client to independently perform personal care ADLs 100% of the time

Physical Therapy
1. Good unilateral standing balance
2. Independent in floor transfers with/without supervision
3. Good static stance with narrow-based quad cane in 2 weeks to enable client to independently perform all personal ADLs

---

procedures and activities the client can safely carry out at home. It should also specify the frequency, amount, and duration of each activity and procedure as well as the degree of supervision and/or assistance that will be required to help the client to carry out the home program safely and accurately.

Examples of treatment procedures for speech-language pathology include: (1) word retrieval exercises, (2) reading comprehension exercises at the four-paragraph level, (3) written expression exercises at the two-paragraph level, (4) home safety problem-solving exercises, (5) self-planning, construction and use of daily planner, and (6) home program for exercises one through five.

Examples of treatment procedures for physical therapy include: (1) weight shifting in sit and stand positions, (2) motor control and muscle reeducation, (3) right upper and lower extremity gait training, (4) cognitive awareness of loss of balance cues, (5) training in recognition and problem-solving pedestrian safety hazards in and out of home, and (6) home program for procedures one through four.

Examples of treatment procedures for occupational therapy include: (1) right upper extremity strength and coordination exercises, (2) visual perceptual training, (3) self-care ADL training, (4) meal preparation training, (5) home program for the above four procedures.

Family Training Goals. These goals identify the training the family will receive to facilitate the application and supervision of the client's home program and to help the client maintain or enhance the abilities achieved from rehabilitation. Examples of family training goals include the following:

1. Spouse and aide will accurately cue client to complete home program 100 percent of the time in two weeks.
2. Spouse and aide will accurately cue client to use pillbox to safely take medications 100 percent of the time in four weeks.
3. Spouse and aide will use correct handling technique during ambulation 100 percent of the time in two weeks.
4. Spouse and aide will be able to identify correct rest position of lower back, leg, and arm to reduce pain 100 percent of the time in two weeks.
5. Spouse and aide will correctly reverse demonstrate right upper extremity exercise program 100 percent of the time in two weeks.
6. Spouse and aide will correctly reverse demonstrate correct right upper extremity protection techniques 100 percent of the time in two weeks.
7. Spouse and aide will provide the correct methods and amount of assistance for upper and lower body dressing 100 percent of the time in three weeks.

What Frequency and Duration of Treatment Will Be Required? This is the seventh and last question regarding medical necessity. The frequency and duration of treatment should be commensurate with the severity of the client's condition as described in the initial evaluation. The content here should also indicate the expected step down in the frequency of treatment across the entire course of treatment. Examples include:

- Physical therapy: three times a week for two weeks, then two times a week for two weeks

- Occupational therapy: three times a week for three weeks, then two times a week for three weeks
- Speech-language pathology: three times a week for three weeks, then two times a week for three weeks

The content of the discharge plan should reflect actions that will be taken before discharge that will act to support and maintain a client's outcome after discharge from rehabilitation. For example:

1. Complete driving evaluation
2. Attend Comebackers Club (a stroke support group)
3. Refer to Mall Walkers Club to maintain endurance and socialization
4. Join senior community center for socialization opportunities
5. Determine if client wants to do volunteer work and, if he or she does, identify type of volunteer work preferred and facilitate contact with facility

PUTTING IT ALL TOGETHER TO ESTABLISH MEDICAL NECESSITY

Up to this point, the content of the initial evaluation report has been presented in relation to each of the seven questions for which responses are needed in order to establish the medical necessity of treatment. The following initial evaluation and treatment plan examples will present this information as it would appear on an actual report.

Speech-Language Pathology: Initial Evaluation and Treatment Plan Content

Medical History. Patient incurred left CVA on 1/28/98. CT on 1/29/98 showed left frontal-temporo infarction. Client has a reactive depression and a premorbid history of hypertension and dizziness.

Prior Level of Function. Prior to CVA, patient was able to communicate all personal, household, community access, and leisure ADL needs.

Current Level of Function. Currently, the patient requires moderate assistance to communicate his personal and household needs and maximum assistance to communicate his community access and leisure needs.

Assessment Results. Client presents with moderate dyspraxia; moderate written language impairment; and moderate attention, short-term memory, and problem-solving impairments.

Expected Outcome. Within 24 visits, the client will be independent in communicating all personal ADL needs, will need standby assistance in communicating household ADL needs, and minimal assist to communicate community ADL needs.

Short-Term Goals. Within 3 weeks, the client will:

1. increase accuracy of confrontation naming to 60% to enable him to communicate personal ADL needs with minimal assistance
2. increase written expression at 3–4 word sentence level to 75% accuracy to enable him to write cards and brief notes with minimal assistance
3. increase accuracy of content and use of daily planner to 75% to enable him to remember and follow his daily routine and manage medications with minimal assistance

Within 6 weeks, the client will:

1. increase accuracy of confrontation naming to 90% to enable him to communicate personal ADL needs with standby assistance.
2. increase written expression accuracy at 2-paragraph level to 90% to enable him to write letters and fill out forms with standby assistance
3. increase accuracy of content and use of daily planner to 90% to enable him to remember and follow his daily routine and manage medications with standby assistance.

Treatment. (1) word retrieval exercises, (2) written expression exercises at the 2-paragraph level, (3) self-planning, construction and use of daily planner, and (4) home program for items 1–3.

Frequency and Duration of Treatment. 3 times a week for 3 weeks, then 2 times a week for 3 weeks.

Family Training Goals. (1) Wife and aide will accurately cue client to complete home program 100% of the time in 2 weeks; and (2) wife and aide will accurately cue client to use pillbox to safely take medications 100% of the time in 4 weeks.

Discharge Plan. Client will attend Comebackers Club (a stroke support group) and join senior community center for socialization opportunities.

Physical Therapy Initial Evaluation and Treatment Plan Content

Patient Name: George Smith
Medical record #: 444092

Diagnostic: CVA
Onset Date: 1/28/98
Admit Date: 2/2/98

Medical History. Client incurred right CVA on 1/28/98. CT on 1/29/98 showed right temporo-occipital infarction. Client presents with left hemiplegia and has a reactive depression and a premorbid history of hypertension and dizziness.

Prior Level of Function. Prior to CVA, patient was independent in all personal, household, community access, and leisure ADLs.

Current Level of Function. Currently, the patient requires moderate assistance for his personal and household ADLs and maximum assistance for his community access and leisure ADLs.

Assessment Results. Patient presents with: (1) mild decrease in left upper and lower extremity strength, (2) poor dynamic standing balance, and (3) a moderate decrease in upper and lower extremity control secondary to moderate proprioceptive impairment.

Expected Outcome. Within 15 visits, the client will be able to ambulate safely with a single-point cane on all surfaces in order to be modified independent in all personal ADLs, with a decreased type and amount of his usual and customary household, community access, and leisure ADLs.

Short-Term Goals. Within 3 weeks, the client will:

1. increase dynamic standing balance and lower extremity strength from poor to fair in order to be minimum assistance in:
   a. ambulating safely with a quad cane on even surfaces
   b. safely ascending and descending 2 stairs with a quad cane and handrail
   c. safely performing toilet, tub, and car transfers
2. increase awareness of balance impairment from poor to fair+ in order to correct for loss of balance with minimal assistance when retrieving objects from high and low cupboards

Within 6 weeks, the client will:

1. increase dynamic standing balance and lower body strength from poor to fair+ in order to be modified independent in:
   a. ambulating safely with a single cane on even and uneven surfaces
   b. safely ascending and descending 6 stairs with a single-point cane and no handrail
   c. safely performing toilet, tub, and car transfers
2. increase awareness of balance impairment from fair+ to good+ in order to correct independently for loss of balance when retrieving objects from high and low cupboards

Treatment. (1) Weight shifting in sit and stand positions, (2) motor control and muscle reeducation, (3) right upper and lower extremity gait training, (4) cognitive awareness of loss of balance cues, (4) training in recognition and problem-solving pedestrian safety hazards in and out of home, (5) home exercise program.

Frequency and Duration of Treatment. 3 times a week for 2 weeks, then 3 times a week for 2 weeks.

Family Training Goals. (1) Wife and aide will use correct handling technique during ambulation 100% of the time in 2 weeks, and (2) wife and aide will be able to identify correct rest position of lower back, leg, and arm to reduce pain 100% of the time in 2 weeks.

Discharge Plan. Client will be referred Mall Walkers Club to maintain endurance and socialization, and will be referred to community aquatics program.

Occupational Therapy: Initial Evaluation and Treatment Plan Content

Medical History. Client incurred right on CVA 1/28/98. CT on 1/29/98 showed left frontal-temporo parietal infarction. Client presents with right hemiplegia and has a reactive depression. Premorbid history of hypertension, dizziness, chronic obstructive pulmonary disease, and peptic ulcer.

Prior Level of Function. Prior to CVA, patient was independent in all personal, household, community access, and leisure ADLs.

Current Level of Function. Currently the patient requires moderate assistance for his personal and household ADLs and maximum assistance for his community access and leisure ADLs.

Assessment Results. (1) Poor right upper extremity strength and coordination, (2) poor right upper extremity sensation, (3) right visual neglect, and (4) poor functional endurance.

Expected Outcome. Within 16 visits, the client will be: (1) modified independent in personal and household ADLs, and (2) standby assistance for community and leisure ADLs.

Short-Term Goals. Within 3 weeks, the client will:

1. maintain F+ sitting posture to be standby assist in grooming
2. increase dynamic sitting balance to F+ to be standby assist in bathing, toileting, and lower body dressing 75% of the time with verbal cues
3. increase bilateral shoulder flexion to 90 degrees to be standby assist for upper body dressing
4. increase right upper extremity coordination to F– to be minimal assist to write legibly
5. exhibit F+ judgment to be standby assist to recognize safety risks during all ADLs and take appropriate precautions

Within 6 weeks, the client will:

1. maintain G+ sitting posture to be modified independent in grooming
2. increase dynamic sitting balance to G+ to be modified independent in bathing, toileting, and lower body dressing 95% of the time without verbal cues
3. increase bilateral shoulder flexion to 90 degrees to be modified independent for upper body dressing
4. increase right upper extremity coordination to F– to be standby assist to write legibly
5. exhibit G+ judgment to be modified independent to recognize safety risks during all ADLs and take appropriate precautions

Treatment. (1) Right upper extremity strength and coordination exercises, (2) visual perceptual training, (3) self-care ADL training, (4) meal preparation training, (5) home program for 1–4.

Frequency and Duration of Treatment. 3 times a week for 3 weeks, then 2 times a week for 3 weeks.

Family Training Goals. (1) Wife and aide will correctly reverse demonstrate right upper extremity exercise program 100% of the time in 2 weeks, (2) wife and aide will correctly reverse demonstrate correct right upper extremity protection techniques 100% of the time in 2 weeks, (3) wife and aide will provide the correct methods and amount of assistance for upper and lower body dressing 100% of the time in 3 weeks.

Discharge Plan. (1) Complete driving evaluation, provide department of motor vehicle contact and refer to physician for medical clearance to drive, (2) determine if client wants to do volunteer work, and, if he does, identify type of volunteer work he prefers and facilitate contact with facility.

Medical Necessity as Seen Through the Eyes of a Medical Reviewer

The previous sections have looked at the development of a report that establishes the medical necessity for treatment from the perspective of the therapist. This section will present the manner in which a medical reviewer evaluates the content of the therapist's report to determine if the medical necessity of treatment has, in fact, been established. The medical reviewer may be the managed care organization's case manager, the provider's internal utilization review staff, a Medicare reviewer seeking to determine whether the bill for services rendered should be paid, or a Medicaid reviewer who is asked to provide prior approval for treatment. In general, all reviewers follow a similar procedure. First, the initial evaluation report is reviewed for technical compliance in relation to the following questions:

1. Is all required case identification and demographic information provided?
2. Is there an acceptable medical diagnosis?
3. Is there an acceptable therapy diagnosis (e.g., impairments caused by the medical condition)?
4. Is there a stated outcome?
5. Are short-term goals stated?
6. Is there a plan of treatment?
7. Is the estimated frequency and duration of treatment stated?

Sometimes, the technical review is either done by computer or manually by a clerk. If the report passes the technical review, a medical professional then reviews it for medical necessity. The medical reviewer usually poses the following four questions when reading the report:

1. Given the medical diagnosis, the type and severity of the client's impairments and handicap, the expected outcome, the goals, and treatment plan, is treatment reasonable and necessary to the client's condition? (i.e., is the client so severely impaired that it is unlikely that significant practical improvement will occur? Is the client so minimally impaired that he or she is not disabled within the context of the demands of the natural environment?)
2. Given the medical diagnosis, the type and severity of the client's impairments and handicaps, the expected outcome, the goals, and treatment plan, is there a reasonable expectation that the client will improve significantly in a reasonable amount of time?
3. Given the medical diagnosis, the type and severity of the client's impairments and handicaps, the expected outcome, the goals, and treatment plan, is the treatment plan specific and effective to the client's condition?
4. Given the medical diagnosis, the type and severity of the client's impairments and handicaps, the expected outcome, the goals, and treatment plan, is the frequency and duration of treatment reasonable to the client's condition?

Establishing the Medical Necessity for Continued Treatment

The therapist must not only provide documentation that substantiates the need to initiate treatment, but also must establish the medical necessity of continued treatment once it has begun. The medical necessity for continued treatment is based on three clinical questions:

1. Is the client making significant practical improvement?
2. Does the client require skilled therapy services to continue to make significant practical improvement?
3. Does the client continue to require the same frequency and duration of treatment?

Progress Report

The content of the therapist's initial evaluation report is used to substantiate the medical necessity of initiating treatment and establishes the plan of treatment as well as identifies the baseline level of severity of the client's impairments, functional limitations, and disabilities. The *progress report* forms the basis for the therapist's and other interested parties' decisions as to whether continued treatment is medically necessary. This determination is made by comparing the client's level of function at the time of the current progress report with his or her level of function documented in the previous progress report as well as his or her baseline level of function that is documented in the therapist's initial evaluation report. The sole basis for the medical necessity of continued treatment is that the comparison of the client's level of function at these three points in time indicate that the client has made significant practical improvement (see Chapter 5). In essence, significant practical improvement is reflected in the client's continued and sustained progress through the three phases of rehabilitation (i.e., impairment reduction, functional limitation reduction, disability reduction) as defined by the National Commission on Medical Rehabilitation and Research (NCMRR) model of rehabilitation (see Exhibit 8–2), which was discussed in Chapter 4.[4]

In the context of the NCMRR model, significant practical improvement is demonstrated when the comparison of the previous and current levels of function indicate either that treatment has reduced the client's level of impairment to such a degree that there has been a commensurate decrease in his or her functional limitations or that the client's functional limitations have been reduced to such a degree that there has been a commensurate decrease in his or her level of disability. A measurable reduction in a client's level of impairments alone does not substantiate the presence of significant practical improvement. Significant practical improvement is demonstrated when the documentation indicates that treatment has resulted in a reduction of either a client's functional limitations or disabilities. In essence, then, a progress report is the therapist's evaluation of the effectiveness of his or her treatment plan.

Progress Report Documentation Guidelines

A progress report should accomplish the following objectives:

- Document the length of time the client has received treatment.
- Document the number of treatments provided.
- Compare the client's current level of function with his or her expected outcome level of function.

Exhibit 8–2 National Commission on Medical Research and Rehabilitation Model of Rehabilitation

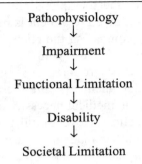

Pathophysiology
↓
Impairment
↓
Functional Limitation
↓
Disability
↓
Societal Limitation

- *Pathophysiology:* The interruption of, or interference with, normal physiological and developmental processes and structures (e.g., stroke, traumatic brain injury, and spinal cord injury).
- *Impairment:* The loss or abnormality of cognitive, emotional, or physiological function, or anatomical structure.
- *Functional Limitation:* Any restriction or lack of ability to perform an action in the manner consistent with the purpose of an organ or organ system.
- *Disability:* An inability or limitation in performing tasks, activities, and roles.
- *Societal Limitation:* Restrictions caused by structural or attitudinal barriers that limit fulfillment of roles or deny access to services and opportunities.

- Compare the client's current status for each short-term goal with the expected status stated in each one. While all short-term goals are usually addressed within each treatment session, therapists often only document in relation to those goals that were particularly emphasized. This results in documentation that gives the appearance that the therapist is jumping from one treatment area to another without bringing sustained changes in any of them. This type of documentation creates the appearance of maintenance care, and conveys the sense that the therapist is not following his or her own treatment plan.
- Use the same forms of measurement that were used in the short-term goal statement when comparing current with previous status for each goal. Shifting from one form of measurement to another fails to

provide the basis for an objective comparison and measurement of current and previous status.

- State new or revised short-term goals in the same terminology and form of measurement as used in the other short-term goals.
- Describe application of any assistive/adaptive equipment, orthotics, and/or prosthetics. Identify the client's response to them and any problems and the actions taken to resolve them. Describe instructions to nursing, family, and/or client regarding their use and indicate whether they were fabricated, sold, rented, or loaned.
- Explain the clinical reason for slow progress, no progress, or regression in level of function and the actions taken to address the reason.
- Explain the clinical reason for any change in diagnosis, expected outcome, and/or treatment plan.
- Report progress toward family training goals.
- Report progress toward discharge plans.

Treatment Note

A therapist is required to enter a treatment note in the client's chart every time the client is seen for treatment. A treatment note, however, is not the same as a progress report. The primary purpose of a treatment note is to provide evidence that the client was treated on a particular day. This information is of considerable importance when there is a question about the amount of a client's bill or in legal proceedings. A treatment note should indicate whether the client was seen on the scheduled date and, if not, why not. It should describe the activities, procedures, and/or modalities employed as well as any assistive or adaptive equipment, orthotics, or prosthetics used. While it is not a progress report, the *treatment note* should reflect the client's general response to treatment during the treatment session as well as anything unusual that may have occurred.

Discharge Report

The discharge report is the final step in establishing the medical justification of continued treatment. In essence, a discharge report is the client's final progress report. Its content should compare the client's functional status at the time of discharge with his or her functional status prior to treatment. To accomplish this, the discharge report compares, in measurable terms, the client's impairments and disabilities both at the time of the initial evaluation and at the time of discharge from treatment. The discharge report should also contain content that describes, in measurable terms, the family education and training goals that were achieved as well as recommendations for postdischarge resources required to sustain the client's outcome after discharge from treatment.

HOW TO WRITE SHORT-TERM GOALS

The short-term goal is the critical link in the chain of clinical case management activities. Regardless of differences among clients and the focus of the different disciplines, all short-term goals should be written in the same format by all disciplines and therapists. Uniformity of documentation is essential to ensure:

- ability of all team members to understand conference progress reports
- clarity and ease of team problem solving
- clarity and uniformity of the team progress report
- speed and ease of team progress report preparation by case manager
- ease of recognizing and understanding client progress by payer case manager
- speed and ease of processing and payment of claims by payer

Structure and Content of Short-Term Goal

A *short-term goal* is a measurable and time-framed description of what the therapist intends to treat and the functional results he or she expects to occur as a product of that treatment. Within this context, a short-term goal is a two-part cause and effect statement.

The cause is represented by a statement that identifies the impairment or functional limitation the therapist will treat and the measurable amount of change the therapist expects to occur in the impairment or functional limitation. The effect is represented by a statement that identifies the measurable improvement in the client's functional performance that the therapist expects to occur as a result of the reduction of the impairment or functional limitation.

The Three Phases of Rehabilitation

The approach to writing short-term goals presented in the following material is based on the expectations of the NCMRR model described earlier in this chapter and in Chapter 4. Specifically, short-term goals should reflect the intent to facilitate a client's progress either from the impairment phase of rehabilitation through the functional limitation phase or from the functional limitation phase through the disability phase of rehabilitation. Within this context, the structure and content of a short-term goal will depend upon the client's phase of rehabilitation and the goal of that phase. Below are listed the three phases of rehabilitation and the standard goal for each phase:

1. Impairment reduction
   Goal: Reduce the degree of an impairment in order to reduce the degree of a functional limitation
2. Functional limitation reduction
   Goal: Reduce the degree of a functional limitation in order to reduce the degree of a disability
3. Disability reduction
   Goal: Further reduction of the disability to enable the client to perform personal, household, community, work, and/or leisure ADLs

Short-Term Goal Formats

Short-term goal formats describe how the cause and effect relationship of a short-term goal should be laid out. The following material will present short-term goal formats, "fill in the blank" model formats, and example short-term goals for the impairment, functional limitation, and disability reduction phases of rehabilitation. This section will conclude with a description of how to select the appropriate type (e.g., impairment reduction, functional limitation reduction, or disability reduction) of short-term goal.

Impairment Reduction Short-Term Goal Format

1. A statement that describes the impairment that you intend to reduce
2. A statement of the degree to which you will reduce the impairment

3. A statement of the amount of time it will take you to reduce the impairment
4. A statement of the functional limitation that will be reduced as a result of the reduction of the impairment
5. A statement of the degree to which the functional limitation will be reduced

A model format for an impairment reduction short-term goal is:

Increase/decrease (statement of the impairment) by (x amount) in (x number of) weeks to enable the client to (statement of the functional limitation) with (x amount) of assistance.

Examples of impairment reduction short-term goals are:

Physical Therapy. Increase right lower extremity (RLE) strength to fair in two weeks to enable client to stand for one minute with standby assistance.

Occupational Therapy. Increase right-hand grip strength to 8 lbs. in two weeks to enable client to pick up small objects with minimum assistance 80 percent of the time.

Speech Pathology. Increase oral-motor sequencing of trisyllabic phoneme strings to 90 percent accuracy in two weeks to enable client to produce three to four unrelated words with minimal assistance.

Functional Limitation Reduction Short-Term Goal Format

1. A statement that describes the functional limitation you intend to reduce
2. A statement that describes the degree to which you will reduce the functional limitation
3. A statement of the time it will take you to reduce the functional limitation
4. A statement of the disability that will be reduced as a result of the reduction of the functional limitation

A model format for a functional limitation reduction short-term goal is:

Increase (statement of the functional limitation that will be reduced) to (x amount) of assistance in (x number of) weeks to enable client to (statement of the disability that will be reduced) with (x amount of) assistance.

Examples of functional limitation reduction short-term goals are:

Physical Therapy. Increase stand to sit and sit to stand transfers to minimal assistance in two weeks to enable client to get on and off the toilet with minimal assistance.

Occupational Therapy. Increase ability to hold and manipulate adaptive feeding instruments to 15 minutes in two weeks to enable client to self-feed with standby assistance.

Speech Pathology. Increase ability to produce three to four word phrases to 90 percent accuracy in four weeks to enable client to describe his or her health care needs in a structured environment with minimal assistance.

Disability Reduction Short-Term Goal Format

1. A statement that describes the disability that will be reduced
2. A statement that describes the degree to which the disability will be reduced
3. A statement that describes the amount of time required to decrease the disability

A model format for a disability reduction short-term goal is:

The client will be able to (statement of the disability that will be reduced) (statement of the degree of disability reduction) in (x number of) weeks.

Examples of disability reduction short-term goals are as follow:

Physical Therapy. Client will be able to get on/off the toilet and in/out of chair or couch independently in two weeks.

Occupational Therapy. Client will be able to self-feed independently at home and in restaurants in two weeks.

Speech Pathology. Client will be able to communicate health care needs independently to his or her physician in four weeks.

Formats for Short-Term Goals That Cover More Than One Functional Limitation/Disability

Frequently, a single impairment will cause multiple functional limitations or disabilities. A short-term goal may only address one impairment; however, a short-term goal may address multiple functional limitations/disabilities that are caused by that impairment. Examples include the following:

Physical Therapy
- Impairment: Decreased left and right hip strength
- Short-Term Goal: Increase strength of left hip flexion to 4 and right hip flexion to 4– in two weeks to enable client to perform personal and household ADLs with minimum assistance.

Occupational Therapy
- Impairment: Decreased left upper extremity (UE) sensory awareness
- Short-Term Goal: Increase ability to judge left UE position, direction and speed of motion, and temperature to 90 percent accuracy in four weeks to enable client to be safe in bathing and kitchen activities with minimal assistance.

Speech Pathology
- Impairment: Decreased short-term memory
- Short-Term Goal: Increase use of memory device to 90 percent of time with 75 percent accuracy in four weeks to enable client to plan and follow daily schedule, remember important household events, and communicate needs to physician with minimal assistance.
- Impairment: Decreased selective attention
- Functional limitations include impaired ability to: (1) maintain consistent behavioral response during a continuous activity, (2) retrieve and hold information for the length of time required to accomplish a task, and (3) keep thoughts in a logical sequential order
- Short-Term Goal: Increase selective attention to 15 minutes in four weeks to enable client to maintain a consistent response during a continuous activity with minimal assistance; retrieve and remember information long enough to complete a task with moderate assistance, and keep thoughts in a logical sequential order with maximum assistance.

How To Select Appropriate Type of Short-Term Goal

The type of short-term goal selected is determined by the client's phase of rehabilitation. Some clients enter rehabilitation at the impairment reduction phase and progress through all three phases. In such cases, the therapist begins with impairment reduction short-term goals, switches to functional limitation goals, and then shifts to disability reduction short-term goals as the client progresses through each phase. Other clients may enter rehabilitation at the functional limitation phase. In those cases, the therapist begins with functional limitation short-term goals and moves to disability goals when the client progresses into the disability phase of rehabilitation. Finally, some clients may be at more than one phase of rehabilitation at the same time. In this instance, the therapist may write an impairment reduction goal for one impairment, a functional limitation goal for another, and a disability short-term goal for yet another impairment depending on the client's level of progress.

A client's phase of rehabilitation is determined by three factors: (1) the general goal the therapist believes the client can attain at any given point in time, (2) the treatment focus that the therapist believes is required to reach that goal, and (3) the type of intervention required to reach that goal.

Impairment Reduction Phase

Goal. Reduce the degree of an impairment in order to reduce the degree of functional limitation.

Treatment Focus. Reduce or compensate for a loss, impairment, or abnormality of a physical, physiologic, and/or neurologic structure or function.

Type of Treatment. Hands-on treatment. This phase of rehabilitation requires the highest frequency and intensity of hands-on facilitation, structure, cues, and immediacy of feedback from the therapist in order to ensure progress toward the goal.

Functional Limitation Phase

Goal. Reduce or compensate for impaired skills that are associated with impaired physical, physiologic, and/or neurologic structure or function.

Treatment Focus. Continued reduction of impairments in the context of tasks that afford the client the opportunity to compare intended actions with achieved results and make appropriate self-corrections with minimal to standby assistance.

Type of Treatment. Coaching and guiding. This phase of rehabilitation is a combination of some direct treatment and coaching the client through the performance of tasks. In this phase, the client's performance of the task is the primary treatment medium rather than direct facilitation provided by the therapist. The client now requires less intense hands-on facilitation and fewer cues, structure, and immediate feedback from the therapist to sustain progress toward the short-term goals.

Disability Reduction Phase

Goal. Resume personal roles within the family and community by enabling the client to perform personal, household, community, work, and/ or leisure activities of daily living.

Treatment Focus. Performance of actual daily living activities to establish the competencies and confidence required to carry them out in the client's daily living environment.

Type of Treatment. Empowerment. This phase of rehabilitation requires the least frequency and intensity of direct therapist intervention. In this phase, the client's performance of the actual daily living tasks, both within the treatment program and at home or in the community, is the singular treatment medium. The client receives the necessary tools to accomplish the tasks and the therapist provides general supervision and feedback to further stabilize and enhance the client's ability to self-monitor and self-correct.

Preparing To Write a Short-Term Goal

The following five-step template can help organize the process of writing a cause and effect short-term goal:

Step 1. Identify the type of short-term goal that is needed.
What am I going to reduce?

a) an impairment_____ or b) a functional limitation _____
or c) a disability _____
Step 2. What is the specific impairment, functional limitation, or disability I intend to reduce?_____
Step 3. To what degree will I reduce it?_____
Step 4. What will the client be able to do when the impairment, functional limitation, or disability is reduced?_____
Step 5. How long will it take to reduce the impairment, functional limitation, or disability?_____

The following examples of short-term goals related to each discipline can be used to practice filling in the blanks in this five-step process.

Speech Pathology

1. *Impairment Reduction Short-Term Goal*
   Increase oral-motor sequencing ability to 90 percent accuracy in four weeks to enable client to produce three to four unrelated words with 25 percent assistance.
2. *Functional Limitation Short-Term Goal*
   Increase ability to produce three to four word phrases to 90 percent accuracy in four weeks to enable client to describe health care needs in a structured environment with 25 percent assistance.
3. *Disability Reduction Short-Term Goal*
   Increase ability to produce two to three connected four-word phrases to 90 percent accuracy in unstructured environments in four weeks to enable client to independently describe his or her health needs.

Physial Therapy

1. *Impairment Reduction Short-Term Goal*
   Increase RLE strength to fair in two weeks to enable client to stand for one minute with standby assistance.
2. *Functional Limitation Reduction Short-Term Goal*
   Increase RLE strength to fair+ in two weeks to enable client to ambulate 50 feet with FWW with minimum assist.
3. *Disability Reduction Short-Term Goal*
   Increase RLE strength to good+ in two weeks to enable client to independently perform stand to sit and sit to stand toilet transfers.

Occupational Therapy

1. *Impairment Reduction Short-Term Goal*
   Increase right hand grip strength from 5 to 8 lbs. in two weeks to enable client to pick up small objects 80 percent of the time with minimum assistance.
2. *Functional Limitation Reduction Short-Term Goal*
   Increase ability to pick up and hold small objects for two minutes in two weeks to enable client to manipulate adaptive feeding utensils with standby assistance.
3. *Disability Reduction Short-Term Goal*
   Increase client's ability to manipulate adaptive feeding instruments with 100 percent accuracy in two weeks to enable client to feed self independently.

Combination of Therapies

The following is an example of a single short-term goal that covers multiple functional limitations and disabilities:

Impairment. Moderate decrease in left UE proprioception, stereognosis, and temperature awareness.

Functional Limitation. (1) Moderate assistance to judge position, direction and speed of motion, location of touch on body, and temperature, and (2) moderate assistance to identify objects by touch only.

Disability. Moderate decrease in safety for bathing and kitchen activities.

Short-Term Goal Addressed for Four Weeks. (1) Increased ability to judge left UE position, direction and speed of motion, and water temperature to 90 percent accuracy; (2) increased ability to identify objects by touch to 90 percent accuracy to enable client to be safe in bathing and kitchen skills with minimum assistance.

HOW TO COMPLETE OUTPATIENT MEDICARE REPORT FORMS

The Medicare program is the largest recipient of clinical documentation. Medicare provides two outpatient rehabilitation documentation forms that the therapists may use to document their clinical information: (1) the "Plan of Treatment for Outpatient Rehabilitation" form (Form HCFA-700) (Exhibit 8–3), and (2) the "Updated Plan of Progress for Outpatient Rehabilitation" form (Form HCFA-701) (Exhibit 8–4). Some providers are linked directly to the payer by computer and use a direct electronic data entry system. The direct data entry system is based on a series of "MAPs," (Exhibits 8–5 through 8–8), which are used to document the same information as the hard copy forms. These forms are not discipline-specific and, therefore, can be used by all disciplines to document their clinical information.

The Health Care Financing Administration (HCFA), which administers the Medicare program, does not require therapists to use these forms to document their clinical information. However, if they are not used, it does require therapists to provide the same information that is called for in these two forms. Some providers modify spacing of the Medicare forms to allow more room for certain types of content. This is particularly true for Section 13 of the 700 form and Section 12 of the 701 form. These sections are the areas in which the therapist is to document the client's entire plan of care. Providers who use the direct data entry system cannot modify it. There is less of a need to modify the MAPs, however, because the space allotted to the clinical content areas scrolls forward to accommodate all of the therapist's clinical information.These two Medicare forms and their required content are crucial for the therapist and are presented here for four reasons:

1. Therapists use them frequently.
2. There is considerable misunderstanding among therapists regarding the expected content of each section.
3. Although Medicare does not require the use of these forms for inpatient rehabilitation or home health rehabilitation, it does expect the availability of similar clinical content when requested.
4. Private payers also expect the same type of clinical documentation.

How To Use the Plan of Treatment for Outpatient Rehabilitation (700) Form

The content of the 700 form covers the first 30 days of treatment (Exhibit 8–3). It serves the same purpose as the therapist's initial evaluation report and also serves as the progress report for the first 30 days of treatment.

Exhibit 8–3 Plan of Treatment for Outpatient Rehabilitation—HCFA Form 700

DEPARTMENT OF HEALTH AND HUMAN SERVICES
HEALTHCARE FINANCING ADMINISTRATION

FORM APPROVED
OMB NO 0938-0227

PLAN OF TREATMENT FOR OUTPATIENT REHABILITATION
(Complete for initial claims only)

1. PATIENT'S LAST NAME FIRST NAME M.I.	2. PROVIDER NO	3. HICN

4. PROVIDER NAME	5. MEDICAL RECORD NO. *(Opt)*	6. ONSET DATE	7. SOC. DATE

8.TYPE ❑ PT ❑ OT ❑ SLP ❑ CR ❑ RT ❑ PS ❑ SN ❑ SW	9. PRIMARY DIAGNOSIS *(Pertinent Medical D.X.)*	10. TREATMENT DIAGNOSIS	11. VISITS FROM SOC.

12. PLAN OF TREATMENT FUNCTIONAL GOALS
GOALS *(Short Term)*

OUTCOME *(Long Term)*

PLAN

13. SIGNATURE *(professional establishing POC including professional. designation)*

14. FREQ/DURATION *(e.g. 3/Wk x 4 Wk.)*

I CERTIFY THE NEED FOR SERVICES FURNISHED UNDER THIS PLAN OF TREATMENT AND WHILE UNDER MY CARE   ❑ N/A

15. PHYSICIAN SIGNATURE   16. DATE

17. RECERTIFICATION
FROM   THROUGH   ❑ N/A
18. ON FILE *(Print/type physician's name)*
❑

20. INITIAL ASSESSMENT *(History, medical complications, level of function at start of care. Reason for referral)*

19. PRIOR HOSPITALIZATION
FROM   TO   ❑ N/A

21. FUNCTIONAL LEVEL *(end of billing period)* PROGRESS REPORT   ❑ CONTINUE SERVICES OR   ❑ DC SERVICES

22. SERVICE DATES
FROM   THROUGH

Form HCFA - 700 (9-89)

Source: Reprinted from Department of Health and Human Services, Health Care Financing Administration.

Exhibit 8–4 Updated Plan of Progress for Outpatient Rehabilitation—HCFA Form 701

DEPARTMENT OF HEALTH AND HUMAN SERVICES
HEALTHCARE FINANCING ADMINISTRATION

FORM APPROVED
OMB NO 0938-0227

UPDATED PLAN OF PROGRESS FOR OUTPATIENT REHABILITATION
(Complete for interim to Discharge Claims. Photocopy of HCFA 700 or 701 is required)

1. PATIENT'S LAST NAME FIRST NAME M.I.	2. PROVIDER NO	3. HICN	
4. PROVIDER NAME	5. MEDICAL RECORD NO. *(Opt)*	6. ONSET DATE	7. SOC. DATE
8. TYPE ❏ PT ❏ OT ❏ SLP ❏ CR	9. PRIMARY DIAGNOSIS *(Pertinent Medical D.X.)*	10. TREATMENT DIAGNOSIS	11. VISITS FROM SOC.
❏ RT ❏ PS ❏ SN ❏ SW	12. FREQ/DURATION *(e.g. 3/Wk x 4 Work)*		

13. CURRENT PLAN UPDATE. FUNCTIONAL GOALS *(Specify changes to goals and plan)*
GOALS *(Short Term)*   PLAN

OUTCOME *(Long Term)*

I HAVE REVIEWED THIS PLAN OF TREATMENT AND RECERTIFY A CONTINUING NEED FOR SERVICES. ❏ N/A ❏ DC   14. RECERTIFICATION FROM   THROUGH   ❏ N/A
15. PHYSICIAN'S SIGNATURE   16. DATE   17. ON FILE *(Print/type physician's name)* ❏

18. REASON(S) FOR CONTINUING TREATMENT THIS BILLING PERIOD *(Clarify goals and necessity for continued skilled care)*

19. SIGNATURE *(or name of professional, including professional. designation)*   20. DATE   21. ❏ CONTINUE SERVICES OR ❏ DC SERVICES

22. FUNCTIONAL LEVEL *(at end of billing period - Relate your documentation to functional outcomes and list problems still present)*

23. SERVICE DATES FROM   THROUGH

Form HCFA - 701 (9-89)

Source: Reprinted from Department of Health and Human Services, Health Care Financing Administration.

Exhibit 8–5 Medicare On-Line Data Entry Form: Medical History, Prior Function

```
MAP 1792                    MEDICARE  A  ONLINE  SYSTEM
SC                          THERAPY INFORMATION ENTRY
HIC              NAME                              DISCIPLINE  STATUS
CLAIM FROM      THRU            PROVIDER          SOC              SUBM ST
PAT CNTL                        ONSET     PRIOR HOSP FROM              TO
PHYS UPIN                       REFER DT          SIGN DT
TOT VISITS   FREQ  FREQ PERIOD  DURATION  EST COMPL DT
PLAN ESTAB         PLAN FROM     THRU        MOST RECENT EVENT
SERVICE STAT  CERT STAT  LAST CERT DT
PROF UPIN                  LST                           FIRST          MID
PROF SIGN DT               PROF DESIGNATION
PRIMARY DIAG               TREATMENT DIAG              NARR
PROGNOSIS        PSYCH DRUGS ADM, IM       IV    PO
PSYCH DRUGS NARR

MEDICAL HISTORY/PRIOR FUNCTIONAL LEVEL NARRATIVE  (NEXT 6 LINES)
```

Source: Reprinted from *Medicare Bulletin* #392, 9/11/95, pp. 390–393.

Exhibit 8–6 Medicare On-Line Data Entry Form: Initial Assessment and Functional Goals

MAP 1793

SC　　　　　MEDICARE A ONLINE SYSTEM

HIC　　　　　THERAPY INFORMATION ENTRY

　　　　　DCN　　　　　DISCIPLINE　　　　　STATUS

INITIAL ASSESSMENT NARRATIVE (NEXT 6 LINES)

FUNCTIONAL GOALS NARRATIVE (NEXT 6 LINES)

Source: Reprinted from *Medicare Bulletin* #392, 9/11/95, pp. 390–393.

Exhibit 8-7 Medicare On-Line Data Entry Form: Treatment Plan

MAP 1794

SC   MEDICARE A ONLINE SYSTEM

HIC   THERAPY INFORMATION ENTRY

                 DCN   DISCIPLINE   STATUS

PLAN OF TREATMENT NARRATIVE (NEXT 6 LINES)

CONTINUING TREATMENT NARRATIVE (NEXT 6 LINES)

Source: Reprinted from *Medicare Bulletin* #392, 9/11/95, pp. 390–393.

Exhibit 8–8 Medicare On-Line Data Entry Form: Progress Reporting

MAP 1795

SC

HIC

MEDICARE A ONLINE SYSTEM

THERAPY INFORMATION ENTRY

DCN

DISCIPLINE

STATUS

PROGRESS REPORTING NARRATIVE (NEXT 12 LINES)

Source: Reprinted from *Medicare Bulletin* #392, 9/11/95, pp. 390–393.

Sections 1 through 5 and Sections 8, 13 through 18, and Section 22 of this form contain technical information that is required for client and provider qualification and payment purposes. Sections 6, 7, 9, 10, 12, 20, and 21 provide clinical information related to the determination of the medical necessity for treatment.

The information regarding the use of the 700 form (Exhibit 8–3) is organized in the following manner. Documentation of the technical information will be presented first and clinical documentation second. Corresponding sections of the hard-copy 700 form and the direct data entry MAPs will be identified. The medical necessity criteria relevant to each section will also be identified. Technical sections that are self-evident with respect to their content will not be addressed.

Technical Information

Section 7: SOC (start-of-care) Date

The start-of-care date is the date the client was evaluated. It is not the date the client was admitted to the medical program, unless the client was evaluated on the day of admission.

Section 9: Primary Diagnosis

The primary diagnosis is the medical condition that has caused the client's impairments. For example: CVA (Stroke), TBI (Traumatic Brain Injury), or Parkinson's disease.

Section 10: Treatment Diagnosis

The treatment diagnosis is the primary impairment caused by the client's medical condition; for example, aphasia or right hemiplegia.

Section 11: Visits from SOC

Enter the actual number of visits that have occurred since the start of care. This section is used by the fiscal intermediary to verify the accuracy of the bill. The number of visits that have been billed must match the number of visits shown in this section.

Section 14: Frequency/Duration

Enter the actual frequency and duration of treatment provided to the client for the billing period (month) covered by the report (700 form) you are writing. Examples of frequency and duration of treatment are:

- If the physician had certified 3 x week x 4 weeks and the client was only seen 2 times a week for 4 weeks, the entry would be 2 x week x 4 weeks.
- If the physician had certified 3 x week x 4 weeks and the patient was seen 3 x week x 2 weeks and 2 x week x 1 week and then 3 x week x 1 week, the entry in Section 14 would be as shown in this example.

Note: It is extremely important to use Section 21 of the 700 and Section 22 of the 701 form to explain why the patient was not seen for the certified frequency and/or duration.

Therapists often confuse this section with the frequency and duration of treatment they are asking the physician to certify for the coming month. That information must be placed at the end of the content in Section 21 of Form 700 and Section 22 of Form 701 not in this section.

Section 15: Physician Signature

The Medicare program requires the client's physician to certify the medical necessity of treatment. The physician's initial order to evaluate and treat "certifies" the medical necessity for the first 30 days of treatment. If the client's physician believes the content of the 700 form substantiates the medical necessity for continued treatment, he or she signs this section. Thus, when the physician signs and dates the 700 form, he or she is *recertifying* the need to continue therapy for the *next 30 days.*

Section 17: Recertification

The dates entered in this section are the beginning ("from") and ending ("through") dates for the next 30-day period of treatment that the physician has recertified as medically necessary. For example, suppose the first 30-day period of treatment began on 6/01/98 and ended on 6/30/98. You are now requesting that the physician recertify the medical necessity of treatment for the period beginning 7/01/98 and ending 7/31/98. You would enter 7/01/98 after "From" and 7/31/98 after "Through." The dates for the first 30 days of treatment are entered in Section 22: "From" 6/01/98 and "Through" 6/30/98.

Section 19: Prior Hospitalization

Enter the inclusive dates (first day to discharge [DC] day) of recent hospitalization pertinent to the client's current plan of treatment. Enter N/A if the hospital stay does not relate to the rehabilitation being provided.

Clinical Information

Section 20: Initial Assessment and MAP 1792: Medical History/Prior Functional Level

The information and examples below pertain to content areas of Section 20, Initial Assessment of Form 700 (Exhibit 8–3) and the direct data entry form MAP 1792 (Exhibit 8–5).

Relevant medical necessity criteria for completing these sections include the following:

1. Does the client have a medical condition?
2. Has the medical condition resulted in a decrease in the client's ability to meet his or her usual and customary daily living needs?
3. Has the medical condition resulted in specific impairments that are causing the client's disabilities?
4. Does the client hold a prognosis of making significant practical improvement?
5. Is treatment reasonable and necessary to the client's condition?

The following information would be entered in Section 20 and/or on MAP 1792, as it relates to the above criteria:

- medical history information that is pertinent to the condition being evaluated/treated

- the client's level of functioning prior to the medical episode
- the client's current level of functioning
- impairments
- medications pertinent to the condition being evaluated/treated
- precautions

For example, a client's medical history might read as follows:
Client incurred right CVA on 1/28/98. CT on 1/29/98 showed left frontal-temporo-parietal infarction. Client presents with left hemiplegia and has a reactive depression. Premorbid history of hypertension, dizziness, chronic obstructive pulmonary disease, and peptic ulcer. Hypertension controlled by medication. Close supervision for fall risk due to dizziness. Prior to CVA, client was independent in all personal, household, community access, and leisure activities of daily living. Currently he requires moderate assistance for his personal and household ADLs and maximum assistance for his community access and leisure ADLs.
Assessment results indicate the client has:

- Speech-language pathology example: (1) moderate dysarthria; (2) moderate written language impairment; and (3) moderate attention, short-term memory, and problem-solving impairments
- Occupational therapy example: (1) poor right upper extremity strength and coordination; (2) poor right upper extremity sensation; (3) right visual neglect; and (4) poor functional endurance
- Physical therapy example: (1) mild decrease in left upper and lower extremity strength; (2) poor dynamic standing balance; and (3) a moderate decrease in upper and lower extremity control secondary to moderate proprioceptive impairment

Section 12: Plan of Treatment Functional Goals; MAP 1793: Functional Goals; and MAP 1794: Plan of Treatment

The information and examples below relate to content areas of Section 12, Form 700 (Exhibit 8–3) and to MAPs 1793 and 1794 (Exhibits 8–6 and 8–7).

Relevant medical necessity criteria for completing these sections includes the following:

- Will the client make significant practical improvement (e.g., is the projected outcome level of function significantly above the client's current level of function)?
- Is the treatment specific and effective to the client's condition?
- Do the interventions require the knowledge, skills, and judgment of a therapist?

Outcome (Long-Term Goals). This part of Section 12 indicates whether the client will make significant practical improvement. The skills/abilities that the client is expected to achieve by the time of discharge from treatment should be entered here.

Examples of long-term goals for each discipline are offered below:

- Speech-language pathology: Within 24 visits, the client will be independent in communicating all personal ADL needs, standby assistance in communicating household ADL needs, and minimal assistance to communicate community ADL needs.
- Physical therapy: Within 15 visits, the client will be able to ambulate safely with a single-point cane on all surfaces in order to be modified independent in all personal ADLs and a decreased type and amount of his usual and customary household, community access, and leisure ADLs.
- Occupational therapy: Within 20 visits, the client will be: (1) modified independent in personal and household ADLs, and (2) standby assistance for community and leisure ADLs.

Short-Term Goals. This section indicates whether the treatment is specific and effective to the client's condition, and whether the interventions are skilled in nature. Enter the short-term goals for the first 30-day treatment period.

Examples of short-term goals for each discipline are as follows:

- Speech-language pathology: Within four weeks, the client will: (1) increase accuracy of confrontation naming to 60 percent to enable him to communicate personal ADL needs with minimal assistance, (2) increase written expression accuracy at three–four word sentence level to 75 percent accuracy to enable him to write cards and brief notes with minimal assistance, (3) increase accuracy of content and use of daily planner to 75 percent to enable him to remember and follow his daily routine and manage medications with minimal assistance.

- Physical therapy: Within four weeks, the client will: (1) increase dynamic standing balance and lower extremity strength from poor to fair in order to be minimum assistance in: (a) ambulating safely with a quad cane on even surfaces, (b) safely ascending and descending two stairs with a quad cane and handrail, (c) safely performing toilet, tub, and car transfers; and (2) increase awareness of balance impairment from poor to fair+ in order to correct for loss of balance with minimal assistance when retrieving objects from high and low cupboards.
- Occupational therapy: Within four weeks, the client will: (1) maintain fair+ sitting posture to be standby assistance in grooming; (2) increase dynamic sitting balance to fair+ to be standby assistance in bathing, toileting, and lower body dressing 75 percent of the time with verbal cues; (3) increase bilateral shoulder flexion to 90 degrees to be standby assistance for upper body dressing; (4) increase right upper extremity coordination to fair– to be minimal assistance to write legibly; and (5) exhibit fair+ judgment to be standby assistance to recognize safety risks during all activities of daily living and take appropriate precautions.

Plan. This part of Section 12 outlines the actual treatment plan for the client and addresses the following relevant medical necessity criteria:

- Is the treatment specific and effective to the client's condition?
- Do the interventions require the knowledge, skills, and judgment of a therapist?

The therapist enters specific activities, procedures, and/or modalities. Some examples of these for each discipline are as follows:

- Speech-language pathology: (1) word retrieval exercises, (2) written expression exercises at the two-paragraph level, (3) self-planning, construction, and use of daily planner, and (4) home program for items 1 through 3.
- Physical therapy: (1) weight shifting in sit and stand positions, (2) motor control and muscle reeducation, (3) right upper and lower

extremity gait training, (4) cognitive awareness of loss of balance cues, (5) training in recognition and problem-solving pedestrian safety hazards in and out of home, and (6) home exercise program.
- Occupational therapy: (1) right upper extremity strength and coordination exercises, (2) visual perceptual training, (3) self-care ADL training, (4) meal preparation training, (5) home program for items 1 to 4.

Section 21: Functional Level and MAP 1795: Progress Reporting

Section 21 of Form 700 (Exhibit 8–3) and MAP 1795 (Exhibit 8–8) represent the progress report for the first 30 days of treatment. As such, the information entered is used to substantiate the medical necessity of continued treatment, if that has been requested, by checking the "continue services" box.

Relevant medical necessity criteria include the following:

- Has the client made significant practical improvement?
- Does the client require skilled services?
- Does the client require the same frequency and duration of treatment?

The therapist enters the following information:

- Enter progress toward each short-term goal as stated in 700, Section 12, or MAP 1793: Functional Goals.
- If one did not treat toward a particular short-term goal during the billing period, state reasons why not. If client did not make progress toward a particular short-term goal, state the reasons and problems that will be addressed to facilitate progress.
- Enter progress toward family education and training goals.
- Enter any new short-term goals.
- Enter the clinical rationale for any changes in diagnosis, expected outcome, and/or treatment plan.
- If continued treatment is requested, enter the frequency and duration of treatment the physician is being requested to certify for the next 30-day period.

Examples of progress reporting for each discipline include the following:

- Speech-language pathology: All goals met: (1) Confrontation naming is 60 percent accurate, client communicates personal ADL needs with minimal assistance, (2) written expression accuracy 75 percent at three–four word sentence level, client is able to write cards and brief notes with minimal assistance, and (3) 75 percent content accuracy and use of daily planner, client is able to remember and follow his daily routine and manage medications with minimal assistance. Wife and aide are accurately cueing client to complete home program 100 percent of the time and are accurately cueing him 100 percent of the time to use pillbox to take medications safely.

  New short-term goals: Within four weeks, the client will: (1) increase accuracy of confrontation naming to 90 percent to enable him to communicate personal ADL needs with standby assistance, (2) increase written expression accuracy at two-paragraph level to 90 percent to enable him to write letters and fill out forms with standby assistance, and (3) increase accuracy of content and use of daily planner to 90 percent to enable him to remember and follow his daily routine and manage medications with standby assistance. Recommend continued speech therapy 3 x week x 3 weeks.

- Physical therapy: All goals met: (1) dynamic standing balance and lower extremity strength is fair, client is minimum assistance in: (a) ambulating safely with a quad cane on even surfaces, (b) safely ascending and descending two stairs with a quad cane and handrail, (c) safely performing toilet, tub, and car transfers; and (2) balance is fair+, client corrects for loss of balance with minimal assistance when retrieving objects from high and low cupboards. Wife and aide are using correct handling technique 100 percent of the time during ambulation and are able to identify correct rest position of lower back, leg, and arm to reduce pain 100 percent of the time in two weeks.

  New short-term goals: (1) Increase dynamic standing balance and lower body strength from poor to fair+ in order to be modified independent in: (a) ambulating safely with a single cane on even and uneven surfaces, (b) safely ascending and descending six stairs with a single-point cane and no handrail, (c) safely performing toilet, tub, and car transfers; and (2) increase awareness of balance impairment from fair+ to good+ in order to independently correct for loss of balance when retrieving objects from high and low cupboards. Recommend continued physical therapy 3 x week x 2 weeks.

- Occupational Therapy
  All goals met: (1) sitting posture is fair+, client is standby assistance in grooming; (2) dynamic sitting balance is fair+, client is standby assistance in bathing, toileting, and lower body dressing 75 percent of the time with verbal cues; (3) bilateral shoulder flexion is 90 degrees, client is standby assistance for upper body dressing; (4) right upper extremity coordination is fair–, client is minimal assistance to write legibly; (5) judgment is fair+, client is standby assistance to recognize safety risks during all activities of daily living and take appropriate precautions. Wife and aide are correctly reverse demonstrating right upper extremity exercise program and the correct right upper extremity protection techniques 100 percent of the time. They are providing the correct methods and amount of assistance for upper and lower body dressing 100 percent of the time.

  New short-term goals: Within four weeks, the client will: (1) maintain good+ sitting posture to be modified independent in grooming, (2) increase dynamic sitting balance to good+ to be modified independent in bathing, toileting, and lower body dressing 90 percent of the time without verbal cues, (3) increase bilateral shoulder flexion to 90 degrees to be modified independent for upper body dressing, (4) increase right upper extremity coordination to fair– to be standby assistance to write legibly, (5) exhibit good+ judgment to be modified independent to recognize safety risks during all activities of daily living and take appropriate precautions. Recommend continued occupational therapy 2 x week x 3 weeks.

Evaluation Only

If you only did an evaluation at the end of a 30-day period AND you plan to continue with treatment in the next 30-day period:

1. Complete all sections except Section 21.
2. Enter evaluation only in Section 21.
3. Enter the recommended frequency and duration for which you request physician certification.

If you only did an evaluation at the end of a 30-day period AND do not intend to continue with treatment, complete all sections except Sections 12, 17, and 21. State the reasons for not continuing with treatment in Section 20.

How To Use the Updated Plan of Progress for Outpatient Rehabilitation (701) Form

If a client is seen for treatment beyond the first certified 30-day treatment period, the 701 form is used to document the client's progress as a result of the continued treatment (Exhibit 8–4). The documentation of the client's type and degree of progress is needed to substantiate that the services provided were, in fact, medically necessary. The 701 form documents progress across all subsequent recertified 30-day treatment periods. Instructions for completing the Medicare 701 Form (Exhibit 8–4) follow below. The information is organized by sections, with relevant medical criteria and examples provided for each content area.

Section 11: Visits from SOC

The relevant medical necessity criteria for this section include the following: Has the client made significant practical improvement, as documented in Section 22, in relation to the amount of treatment received to date? Enter the cumulative number of visits completed since services began in Section 11. For example: Mr. Jones began therapy on 6/01/98 and was seen three times a week for four weeks. At the end of four weeks (6/30/98), he had been seen for 12 visits. He continued therapy at three times a week for four weeks from 7/01/98 through 7/31/98. His total number of visits from the start of care is 24, which would be entered into Section 11.

If Mr. Jones did not receive all of the scheduled visits, then enter the actual number received in Section 11 and explain why he didn't receive all scheduled visits in Section 22.

Section 12: Frequency and Duration of Treatment

The relevant medical necessity criterion governing this section is whether the client has made significant practical improvement in relation to the frequency and duration of treatment (e.g., has treatment been reasonable and necessary to the client's condition?).

Enter the frequency and duration of treatment that actually occurred during the 30-day period of treatment covered by the report. If the client did not receive the certified frequency and duration of treatment, explain why in Section 22. Do not enter the frequency and duration of treatment that you are asking the physician to recertify for the next 30-day period.

Section 13: Current Plan Update/Functional Goals; MAP 1793: Functional Goals; and MAP 1794: Plan of Treatment

Relevant medical review criteria to be addressed in Section 13 and in MAPs 1793 and 1974 (Exhibits 8–6 and 8–7) include: Has the client made significant practical improvement? Did the client achieve the majority of his or her short-term goals; have these goals either been modified or new goals added in a manner that indicates the client has the potential to attain an even higher level of function if treatment is continued for another 30 days?

Goals (Short-Term). Enter all short-term goals that were carried over from the previous 30-day treatment period and enter any new short-term goals that were established either at the beginning of or during the current 30-day period. Explain why new short-term goals are added or previous goals are dropped in Section 22.

Outcome (Long-Term). These goals remain the same throughout treatment unless otherwise modified. If they are modified, explain why in Section 22.

Plan. Enter previous treatment plan and any modifications to it. Explain the clinical rationale for any modifications in Section 22.

Section 18: Reasons for Continuing Treatment This Billing Period and MAP 1794: Continuing Treatment

This section is designed to clarify goals and the necessity for continued skilled care.

Relevant medical review criteria are as follow: Services must be reasonable and necessary to the client's condition. Did the type and amount of improvement made by the client during the previous 30-day treatment period indicate that the client would continue to make significant practical improvement if treatment continued during another 30-day period? Did the type and amount of improvement made by the client during the previous 30-day treatment period indicate that skilled services are required to sustain continued improvement?

When completing the client's first 701 report, enter the information from Section 21 of that client's previous 700 report in this section (see Exhibit 8–3). The type and degree of progress made by the client in the first 30-day treatment period, and documented in Section 21 of the 700 form, substantiated the medical necessity for continued treatment into the next 30-day period of treatment. Consequently, the previously reported progress formed the therapist's "reason" for continuing treatment past the first 30-day period. Following are examples for Section 18 content, as it applies to each discipline.

Speech-Language Pathology. All goals met: (1) confrontation naming to 60 percent accuracy, client communicates personal ADL needs with minimal assistance, (2) written expression accuracy 75 percent at three-four word sentence level, client is able to write cards and brief notes with minimal assistance, (3) 75 percent content accuracy and use of daily planner, client is able to remember and follow his daily routine and manage medications with minimal assistance. Wife and aide are accurately cueing client to complete home program 100 percent and are accurately cueing him 100 percent of the time to use pillbox to take medications safely.

New short-term goals: Within four weeks, the client will: (1) increase accuracy of confrontation naming to 90 percent to enable him to communicate personal ADL needs with standby assistance, (2) increase written expression accuracy at two-paragraph level to 90 percent to enable him to write letters and fill out forms with standby assistance, (3) increase accuracy of content and use of daily planner to 90 percent to enable him to remember and follow his daily routine and manage medications with standby assistance.

Physical Therapy. All goals met: (1) dynamic standing balance and lower extremity strength is fair, client is minimum assistance in: (a) ambulating safely with a quad cane on even surfaces, (b) safely ascending and descending two stairs with a quad cane and handrail, (c) safely performing toilet, tub, and car transfers; (2) balance is fair+, client corrects for loss of balance with minimal assistance when retrieving objects from high and low cupboards. Wife and aide are using correct handling technique 100 percent of the time during ambulation and are able to identify correct rest position of lower back, leg, and arm to reduce pain 100 percent of the time in two weeks.

New short-term goals: (1) Increase dynamic standing balance and lower body strength from poor to fair+ in order to be modified independent in: (a) ambulating safely with a single cane on even and uneven surfaces, (b) safely ascending and descending six stairs with a single-point cane and no handrail, (c) safely performing toilet, tub, and car transfers; and (2) increase awareness of balance impairment from fair+ to good+ to in order to independently correct for loss of balance when retrieving objects from high and low cupboards.

Occupational Therapy. All goals met: (1) sitting posture is fair+, client is standby assistance in grooming, (2) dynamic sitting balance is fair+, client is standby assistance in bathing, toileting, and lower body dressing 90 percent of the time without verbal cues, (3) bilateral shoulder flexion is 90 degrees, client is standby assististant for upper body dressing, (4) right upper extremity coordination is fair–, client is minimal assistance to write legibly, (5) judgment is fair+, client is standby assistance to recognize safety risks during all activities of daily living and take appropriate precautions. Wife and aide are correctly reverse demonstrating right upper extremity exercise program and the correct right upper extremity protection techniques 100 percent of the time. They are providing the correct methods and amount of assistance for upper and lower body dressing 100 percent of the time.

New short-term goals: Within four weeks, the client will: (1) maintain good+ sitting posture to be modified independent in grooming, (2) increase dynamic sitting balance to good+ to be modified independent in bathing, toileting, and lower body dressing 100 percent of the time, (3) increase bilateral shoulder flexion to 90 degrees to be modified independent for upper body dressing, (4) increase right upper extremity coordination to fair– to be standby assistance to write legibly, (5) exhibit good+ judgment to be modified independent to recognize safety risks during all activities of daily living and take appropriate precautions.

The information for Section 18 in all subsequent recertified 30-day treatment periods is drawn from Section 22 of the 701 form. The type and degree of progress that is documented in this section at the end of the 30-day period is the therapist's "reason" (i.e., substantiation of medical necessity) for continuing treatment for the next 30-day period.

Section 22: Functional Level and MAP 1795: Progress Reporting

The information and examples below relate to Section 22 of the 701 Form (Exhibit 8–4) and MAP 1795 (Exhibit 8–8).

Relevant medical review criteria include the following: Services must be reasonable and necessary to the client's condition. That is, did the client make significant practical improvement? Did the client require skilled services to achieve the attained improvement? Has the type and degree of improvement brought the client significantly closer to the attainment of the expected outcome?

This section includes:

- progress toward each short-term goal that is stated in Section 13. If you did not treat toward a particular short-term goal during the 30-day period, state why you did not. If the client did not make progress toward a particular short-term goal, state the reasons and what you will do to manage the problems.
- the clinical rationale for any new short-term goals or modifications in expected outcome and/or treatment plan
- progress toward family education/training goals
- the requested frequency and duration of treatment if you are requesting recertification for another 30-day period of treatment

Examples for each discipline are included below.

Speech-Language Pathology. All goals met: (1) confrontation naming accuracy is 90 percent, client able to communicate personal ADL needs with standby assistance, (2) written expression accuracy at two-paragraph level is 90 percent, client able to write letters and fill out forms with standby assistance, (3) content accuracy and use of daily planner is 90 percent, client is able to remember and follow his daily routine and manage medications with standby assistance.

Physical Therapy. All goals met: (1) dynamic standing balance and lower body strength is fair+, client is modified independent in: (a) ambulating safely with a single cane on even and uneven surfaces, (b) safely ascending and descending six stairs with a single-point cane and no handrail, (c) safely performing toilet, tub, and car transfers; and (2) awareness of balance impairment is good+, client independently corrects for loss of balance when retrieving objects from high and low cupboards.

Occupational Therapy. All goals met: (1) sitting posture is good+, client is modified independent in grooming, (2) dynamic sitting balance is good+, client is independent in bathing, toileting, and lower body dressing 100 percent of the time, (3) bilateral shoulder flexion is 90 degrees, client is modified independent for upper body dressing, (4) right upper extremity coordination is fair–, client is standby assistance to write legibly, (5) judgment is good+, client is modified independent to recognize safety risks during all activities of daily living and take appropriate precautions.

CONCLUSION

Managed care has created major changes in the delivery of health care services. As the changes in direct client care unfold, the critical importance of excellent clinical documentation will become clear. The original purpose of clinical documentation was to create a "memory" of the longitudinal health care interventions provided to a client and the client's response to them. Thus, during the early phase of health care, clinical information was documented solely for the purpose of good clinical case management. As health care evolved, documentation became important in a number of different ways, so it became critical to successful reimbursement, licensure, accreditation, and litigation.

Managed health care will now create yet another use for documentation. The clinical and financial information generated by therapists will become a vital corporate resource. Today, the management of health care information and the management of the provider's business are inextricably interrelated and interdependent. In a managed care environment, survival will depend upon a provider's ability to quickly and continuously collect, organize, and manage clinical and financial information. To accomplish this, providers will develop health management information systems that integrate clinical and financial information to manage a client's course of rehabilitation both prospectively and concurrently. Health information systems will empower the team to manage the quality and cost of the services they provide. These systems will provide the team with immediate access to a client's total clinical status and financial resources at any given time in relation to the expected clinical status and financial resources at that time. The clinical and financial data collected and integrated in a health information system will also create the database that will be required to conduct the outcome studies that are necessary to continually improve the effectiveness and efficiency of service delivery. Both therapists and management hold significant responsibilities in this new documentation era. Therapists must understand that what they document is a vital corporate resource and ensure that they provide excellent objective and measurable documentation of their clinical decisions and interventions. The phrase "garbage in—garbage out," often used to describe the usefulness of computer-generated information, is apropos here. The content of this chapter has been directed toward guidelines and methods of generating objective and measurable clinical information, which can be used to make objective clinical case management and business decisions. While therapists are responsible to provide useful clinical and business management information, management is responsible to provide therapists with the tools needed to meet their responsibility. Management must provide therapists with the health information management systems technology that will allow them to carry out their vital documentation role in the least time-consuming manner possible. Management cannot expect "high tech" performance without "high tech" systems.

REFERENCES

1. R. Scott, The Legal Standard of Care, *Clinical Case Management* March/April (1991).
2. R. Harker, *Malpractice and Other Bases of Potential Liability for the Physical Therapist*, 5.1—Risk Management, an APTA, Malpractice Resource Guide (Alexandria, VA: American Physical Therapy Association).
3. S. Ablen, "Importance of Documentation to Patient Care Reimbursement," in *Documenting Functional Outcomes in Physical Therapy*, ed. D. Stewart and S. Ablen (St. Louis, MO: Mosby, 1993), 67.
4. National Advisory Board on Medical Rehabilitation Research, *Draft V: Report and Plan for Medical Rehabilitation Research* (Bethesda, MD: National Institutes of Health, 1992).

SUGGESTED READING

Tan, J. 1995. *Health Management Information Systems: Theories, Methods, and Applications*. Gaithersburg, MD: Aspen Publishers, Inc.

INDEX

A

Accreditation, documentation for, 261
Activity indicators, purpose of, 103
Acute inpatient rehabilitation, level of care, 78
Adapted living, meaning of, 91
Assisted living, meaning of, 91
Audits, and documentation, 264
Authorization, meaning of, 19

B

Balanced Budget Act, 4, 14
Best outcome, elements of, 16
Brainstorming, problem solving, 231, 232
Break-even point, 32–33
Budget, 30–33
   break-even point, 32–33
   cost management, 30–32
   example budget, 31
   operating budget, 32
Business management
   basic concepts, 26
   budget, 30–33
   cost per unit of service, 28–29
   costs, 26–28
   expenses, reduction of, 34–35
   gross revenue, 30
   price of service, 29–30
   productivity, increasing, 35–36
   revenue sources, 37–41
   volume, increasing, 36

C

Capitation, meaning of, 19
Case management

concurrent case management, 133–134, 142–151
   meaning of, 19
   prospective case management, 133, 134–142
   retrospective case management, 134, 151–169
Case manager
   meaning of, 19
   role of, 55
Certification, and documentation, 259
Client management plan
   client/family goals, 98–103
   components of, 136
   critical pathways, individualized, 119–121
   discharge plan, 122–125
   needs-based treatment plan, 103–110
   outcome-driven treatment, 91–98
   prospective case management, 135–142
   resource utilization plan, 118–119
   risk management, 110–118
   short-term goals, 121–122
Client satisfaction
   aspects of, 165–166
   basis of, 165
   outcome studies, 164–167
   survey questions, 195
Clinical case management
   documentation for, 259, 263
   level of care, 75–81
   risk for complications, 81–82
   service delivery format, 64–74
   therapy resources, 47–52
   tools for, 46–47
   treatment duration, 52–63
Coaching, peer coaching, 73–74
Comfort level, and client satisfaction, 166
Communication
   clear communication guidelines, 218–219
   with family members, 191, 193–194

317

medical necessity criteria, 134–135
Prospective payment system (PPS)
  legal aspects, 4
  Medicare PPS, 8–14
  private sector PPS, 7–8
Provider, role of, 20

Q

Quality
  components of, 16
  dimensions of, 46
  outcome studies as measure, 157
Quality of care
  client definition of, 152
  payer definition of, 153
  provider definition of, 153–154
  and retrospective case management,
    152–154

R

Rehabilitation
  best outcome, 16
  NCMRR model, 88–90
  profit as goal, 24–25
  services, types of, 24
  valued outcome, 17
Rehabilitation aides, 70–72
  skilled services, 71
  unskilled services, 71–72
Rehabilitation Institute of Chicago
  Functional Assessment Scale
  (RICFAS), 161
Rehabilitation model, health care, 87
Rehabilitation outcome studies, 158
Rehabilitation process
  process of, 88, 90
  purpose of, 88
Request for services, 101
  example of, 127–130
Resource-based relative value scale
  (RBRVS), 13–14
  work, elements of, 13
Resource management, 47–52
  discipline utilization, 50–52
  modulating frequency of therapy, 52
  only necessary disciplines, 48–50

treatment priority ranking, 51–52
Resource utilization groups (RUGs), 8–12
Resource utilization plan, 118–119
  elements of, 119
  establishing plan, 118–119
Response to disablement, as risk factor,
  111, 114
Retrospective case management, 151–169
  aspects of, 134
  outcome studies, 155–169
  program evaluation, 154–155
  quality of care/value issues, 152–154
Retrospective review, outpatient
  rehabilitation, 56
Revenue sources, 37–41
  indemnity insurance plans, 38
  managed care organizations, 38–39
  Medicaid, 38
  Medicare, 37
  private payments, 39–41
Rights and responsibilities, of clients, 191,
  192–193
Risk, types of, 81, 111
Risk management, 81–82, 110–118
  case example, 112–116
  for diabetes mellitus, 117
  for falls, 116–117
  procedures in, 111
  risk prevention plan, 116–118
  for stroke, 117–118
Risk pool, meaning of, 20

S

Secondary conditions, as risk factor, 111,
  113–114
Self-managed rehabilitation team, 209–242
  clarification of roles/authority, 222–224
  client care role, 215
  communication channels, 224–225
  communication role, 214, 217–219, 221
  concept of team, 213–214
  conflict resolution, 219, 225–228
  definition of, 211
  documentation by, 214–215, 220
  empowerment of, 241–242
  expectations of members, 215–216
  functions of, 210–211, 212–213
  implementation functions of, 239